Kill as Few
Patients as
Possible

Kill as Few Patients as Possible

And Fifty-Six Other Essays
on How to Be the World's
Best Doctor

Oscar London, MD, WBD

TEN SPEED PRESS
Berkeley

All rights reserved. Published in the United States by Ten Speed Press, an imprint
of the Crown Publishing Group, a division of Random House,Inc., New York.
www.crownpublishing.com
www.tenspeed.com

Ten Speed Press and the Ten Speed Press colophon are registered
trademarks of Random House, Inc.

Excerpts from this book appeared in Medical Economics magazine.

Library of Congress Cataloguing-in-Publication Data
London, Oscar
   Kill as few patients as possible.
   1. London, Oscar-Anecdotes. 2. Medicine-Anecdotes, facetiae, satire,etc.
3. Physicians-Anecdotes, facetiae, satire, etc. I. Title.
   R154.L57A3198761086-23107

ISBN: 978-1-58008-917-3

Printed in the United States of America on recycled paper (50% PCW)

Cover design by Ed Anderson
Text design by Tasha Hall

15 14 13 12 11

First Hardcover Edition

To Harold and Lil

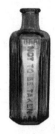

Contents

Warning

IF YOUR PHYSICIAN ASPIRES to be the World's Best Doctor, he or she will have to wait until I die. I am seventy-seven, don't smoke, and always wear my seat belt. I have taken the precaution of descending from ancestors who lived well into their nineties.

I have taken time from my busy—but not killing—practice of internal medicine to pass along some hard-won strategies that, at best, will save your life. Or, at least, will permit your own physician to become the world's *second* best doctor. Then, when Hippocrates and Aesculapius summon me to join their Group Practice in the Sky, your healer will be in the catbird seat. Your shaman will be poised to assume my current role of Mother Earth's Favorite Son—the Doctor. Or Daughter, as the case may be.

How did I get to be Top Doc? How come heads of state phone me long distance, at odd hours, to say they took the two aspirin and now what? Why does my appointment book read like a compendium of *Who's Who*, *Burke's Peerage*, and *People* magazine?

What *is* the key to my success? Is it my uncommon good looks? My uncanny diagnostic skills? My charisma? My modesty? Yes, all of those, but more important: my strict adherence to the rules.

Introduction to the 20th Anniversary Edition

SINCE I WROTE *Kill as Few Patients as Possible* twenty years ago, "a lot of water has been passed," to quote Sam Goldwyn. The past decade has brought about a not-so-bloodless revolution in American medicine known as managed care. The for-profit, publicly traded HMOs have wrested control of your health from Doctors of Medicine and slipped it into the hands of Masters of Business Administration.

The ultimate goal of medicine used to be the enhancement of your physical and emotional well-being, at all costs. Now, it's the enhancement of your HMO's profits at the lowest expenditure for your well-being that they can get away with.

The rules in this book on How to be the World's Best Doctor have required only modest revision to bring them up to date. The HMOs are making it harder for you to see specialists, but your own primary-care doctor can still save your life by mastering my rules and, from time to time, bending your HMO's rules.

The HMOs have cut out a chunk of your doctor's heart and wallet, but so far have left his or her brain intact. Your HMO will try to deny you access to certain high-tech diagnostic and therapeutic tools, but no electronic gizmo can match your doctor's soft, furrowed brain in figuring out what's wrong with you and treating you for it.

With premature death now regarded as a cost-saving outcome under managed care, you need the World's Best Doctor, more than ever, to teach your physician how to kill as few patients as possible.

—*Oscar London, MD, WBD*

Rule 1

Be Jewish

Now IT IS ENTIRELY POSSIBLE—but laughable—to practice internal medicine and not be Jewish. I submit: who else but a Jew has the innate capacity for suffering that can get you through a working day in a medical office? I will say this: if some internists were not lucky enough to be born Jewish, surviving medical school and coping with managed care entitle them to honorary membership in the family of Abraham, Isaac, and Jacob—and Job.

If "Jewish internist" is a redundancy, is "non-Jewish internist" an oxymoron? No. Some of my best and brightest friends are non-Jewish internists.

One of them is Dr. Roy Walker of Fairfax, Iowa. In my third year of medical school, I was farmed out for eight weeks to Dr. Walker, an internist in a small rural town near Cedar Rapids. A short, stocky man, Roy Walker was born to be a third baseman but had somehow gotten sidetracked into medicine. I followed him through his working days and marveled at his ability to field his patients' complaints and then step up and hit diagnostic home runs.

One morning at the local hospital, we visited the bedside of an old Amish blacksmith who was recovering from viral pneumonia. Fifteen of the patient's relatives were jammed into the room. The men were bearded. The women wore no makeup. All were dressed in simple garments the color of Iowa wheat and topsoil. Except for the modern hospital bed it was a scene out of the Old Testament—the Book these people lived by.

Dr. Walker introduced me to every soul in the room, not missing one of their names. When I had shaken the last calloused hand, the old man in the bed stared at me with fire in his eyes.

"That star!" he cried, pointing a trembling, arthritic finger at the gold Mogen David dangling from my neck. "Dr. London, are you a Chew?"

Uh-oh, I thought, my first brush with anti-Semitism and I'm outnumbered sixteen to one.

"Yes, I'm a Jew," I replied, looking him in the eyes.

The room fell silent. "I knew it!" said the old man triumphantly, extending both arms to me. "A Chew!"

The faces around me lit up with smiles of delight and amazement. I was the first living Jew these Fundamentalists had ever seen—a genuine Hebrew, a biblical celebrity! Charlton Heston's Moses was a walk-on part compared to my role as a Jewish medical student in Fairfax, Iowa.

It was necessary for me to shake everyone's hand again. Several of the people reverently touched the sleeves of my short white jacket. Dr. Walker looked crestfallen.

I sometimes regret leaving Iowa for the East Coast. A Jew moving to New York to practice internal medicine is certainly hauling coals to Newcastle. I could have spent my career in Iowa, blissfully reaping adulation each day in the office—an honest-to-God Jew among the honest-to-God Amish.

Rule 2

Have a Lovely Office

MY PATIENTS' TREATMENT BEGINS with my receptionist's smile. A receptionist should not only have a dynamite smile but also radiate perfect health, competence, and serenity. If a male doctor finds a female receptionist with all these traits, it will be necessary for him to fly off with her to Acapulco, leaving his marriage and his practice in a shambles. I tell my younger colleagues, "Try to find a nice receptionist, but don't overachieve."

A doctor's office should be decorated tastefully—but not expensively, unless he prefers a burglar over a janitor to clean up after hours.

To practice world-class medicine, a physician needs a consultation room, three examining rooms, a padded cell, and a restroom. If he's not into padded cells, he can lock himself up from time to time in his consultation room and scream into a throw pillow.

He must not pipe music into his waiting room. If he has a burning desire to inflict music on his patients, he should bring in a live string quartet and restrict the musicians to Haydn and Schubert.

If a physician wants to destroy his practice, he might consider bringing in an accordion player. (One night at a restaurant, I reached out and plunged my dinner knife into the bellows of an approaching accordion; the stricken look on the player's face when the wind was knocked out of his "Lady of Spain" was well worth the price of damages.)

A physician should choose indoor plants for his waiting room carefully. The unseemly bulge in his Venus flytrap might have been his three o'clock appointment.

Rule 3

If You Can't Save Your Patient's Life, Find Someone Who Can

IT's THE YOUNG DEATHS that kill you. If you can save one person from dying young in your entire career, you can feel triumphant when you pull off your stethoscope for the last time. In 1968, one of the coldest fish who ever entered the mainstream of medicine was a sixty-three-year-old hematologist, now dead, who practiced down the hall from me. His dour personality defeated the spirit of hundreds of people who came to him for help. One of these was a gorgeous twenty-four-year-old woman; she had returned, deathly ill, to the States after a stint in Central America with the Peace Corps.

It was I, the World's Best Doctor, who referred this dying woman to the cold fish. She had consulted me at the insistence of her parents. A thorough workup at a famous medical center had left her with a diagnosis of aleukemic leukemia. The parents refused to accept that death warrant; the patient was too sick to care.

When I examined her, I despaired. Her lymph nodes were the size of golf balls; her liver and spleen, soccer balls. I reviewed the results of her previous diagnostic tests in detail. I finally concluded that I didn't know what the hell was wrong with her. At that point, I called in the cold fish.

Dr. Carp (as I will call him) was the brightest physician I'd ever known. He subscribed to, and devoured, sixty medical journals—no issue of which he ever threw away; his consultation room resembled a Times Square magazine stand. I warned the patient and her parents that Dr. Carp would not bowl them over with his personality, but if anyone could put an accurate label on her illness, he could.

The day after I referred her, Dr. Carp called me on the phone. I was startled to detect a hint of animation in his voice as he invited me to look at the patient's bone marrow slide. Leave it to Dr. Carp to repeat a painful bone marrow aspiration on the patient after she had already had two at the medical center. I told my receptionist I'd be down the hall for a few minutes and to hold the fort.

Dr. Carp was seated at his $8,000 dual microscope as I was ushered into his small office laboratory. Without taking his eyes off the microscope, he beckoned me to sit down opposite him and peer into the second pair of eyepieces on the scope.

The bone marrow smear looked a lot like myeloid suppression to me.

"Look at the red cell in the very center of the field," he said. "What do you see next to its left border?"

I looked, feeling like a first-year medical student about to be tossed onto the economy.

"A platelet?" I guessed.

"Uh-uh," said Dr. Carp, switching the lens to a much higher magnification. "Take another look."

And there it was. A tiny one-eyed monster that was killing the patient. "What the hell kind of parasite is *that*?" I asked. The hairs on the back of my neck stood up like exclamation points.

"The amastigote of *Leishmania donovani*," he said, savoring each syllable.

"You son of a bitch," I said, kicking him hard on the shins under the table. "You saved her life."

To soften the blow, I leaned forward and bestowed a loud kiss on the epicenter of his balding pate.

Dr. Carp looked up for the first time from his scope. "Why Oscar," he said, "that was very sweet of you."

The merest trace of a smile was imprinted on his bloodless lips. That smile remained there for the last ten years of his life. The patient's response to high doses of Pentostam was a wonder to behold. She is now in her fifties, a successful author, and an ecstatic mother of three.

Did this case wrest from me the title of World's Best Doctor? Not at all. A clear understanding of how much I don't know about medicine is one of my great strengths.

After practicing medicine intensely for a few decades, what you ultimately learn is the phone number of a cold fish, or a warm heart, who can save your patient's life when you can't.

Rule 4

Don't Call Me "Doctor"; Don't Call Me "Doc"

I BECOME APOPLECTIC WHEN a new receptionist refers to me as "Doctor" instead of "Doctor London."

"Doctor is tied up at the hospital and will be a little late."

"Doctor will see you now."

"Doctor wants you to make another appointment in June."

This reverential use of "Doctor" is a throwback to an age when physicians had little more to offer patients than a megadose of holiness—when an ethereal stench of sanctimony pervaded their offices. "Doctor will be with you in a minute." As far as I'm concerned, the high and mighty "Doctor" has no place in an up-to-date, down-to-earth medical office.

At the risk of sounding stuffy, I must confess to being less than overjoyed when a patient calls me "Doc." I realize that "Doc" is often used as a term of endearment. But to me, "Doc" is what you call an excellent poker player who never went to medical school and what you call the town drunk who did. "Doc" is what Bugs Bunny calls Elmer Fudd. "Doc" also sounds too much like "duck," a species of fowl that goes, "quack-quack." To sum up, "Doctor" is not pleased to be called "Doc."

While we're on the subject, I make a point of addressing PhD's as "Doctor" unless instructed not to. They earned their doctorate; I earned mine. In my neck of the medical woods, there are so many PhD's and physicians per capita that everyone seems to be calling each other "Doctor." A few years ago, I hired a receptionist who had earned a PhD in botany. She once informed me, "Doctor London, Doctor Shapiro's wife, Doctor Gottlieb-Shapiro, is calling you from Doctor Mishkin's office."

"Thank you, Doctor Oglethorpe," I replied to the receptionist.

I had to let her go. She may have had a PhD in botany, but she let all the plants in my office die.

Besides, we were doctoring each other to death.

Rule 5

Keep Eye Contact with Your Receptionists

I CAN'T EMPHASIZE ENOUGH how important it is for a doctor to watch every move his receptionist makes, whether or not she bends like a ballerina. I don't bury myself in a back consultation room. I sit up front where my receptionist can flag me down for an urgent message or beam me a smile when I'm bleeding internally. The receptionist in a doctor's office has too much power to be trusted unobserved. I have watched, in shock, a receptionist direct a critically ill patient to a seat in the waiting room rather than have him come in for an immediate exam. I have listened to a receptionist dispense fatal medical advice over the telephone. ("Why don't you see if some bicarbonate of soda will make that chest pain go away?")

Since she's on the front line of a medical practice, she has the powers of life and death. If the doctor is interred in a back office, she may be tempted to handle his practice like an executor managing the estate of a dearly departed. ("Mrs. Kolodny, Doctor won't be able to see you about your swollen leg until next Thursday.") Like hell I won't!

Through the open door of my consultation room, I also observe whether my receptionist suffers from that most insidious of staff infections, Fear of Filing.

Rule 6

Tell an Addict to Take a Walk

I WILL AGREE TO treat just about anyone who appears at my office door—but never an addict. My policy on accepting new patients is taken from the poem on the Statue of Liberty: "Give me your tired, your poor, your huddled masses yearning to breathe free." Huddled masses yearning to breathe free—that's my waiting room on a Friday afternoon. The Statue of Liberty, as far as I can tell, is not carrying a torch for an addict and neither am I.

The day I started practice I resigned from the first case I saw. An angelic, middle-aged man limped piteously into my office. For a half hour I listed to his convoluted story about a severe, chronic pain in the first three toes of his right foot. At the conclusion of his heart-breaking narrative, he looked down at his open-toed tennis shoe and wondered if I'd write him a prescription for aspirin with codeine. I promptly asked him to take a walk, his limp notwithstanding, and find another doctor. Any patient who requests a narcotic prescription on his first visit is out my door before you can say Vicodin.

For years I tried to rehabilitate a wealthy married couple who were hooked on vodka. At breakfast they tinged their vodka with orange juice; at lunch, they pinkened their vodka with tomato juice; at dinner, they sweetened their vodka with vodka. Each year at Christmas they were found sprawled face down in the snow outside their front door. They consistently won the yuletide lawn decoration award in their neighborhood and were a nightmare to care for.

I finally resigned from their case. They understood completely and even drank to my health. That New Year's Eve they spent under the care of their new doctor—in the hospital.

Show me a young, beautiful cocaine addict and I will show her the door. As she stands out in the cold with the wind whistling through her nose, I point over her shoulder and say, "Get out of town and find some place where you can't buy the stuff."

The codeine junkie, the alcoholic, the slave to cocaine all need doctors, all right—but not in private practice.

I instruct my receptionist to screen them out when they call for their first appointment. I have her on the alert for slurred speech, the sound of gunfire in the background, a faint whistle in the foreground. If a junkie escapes her net and I find myself face-to-face or nose-to-nose with one of these Doctor Destroyers, I politely suggest, "I'm afraid I'm not the kind of doctor who can help you. Let me give you the names of some clinics that might be able to treat you."

If the addict still won't budge from the office, I have no choice but to press the button that activates the trapdoor beneath the patient's chair.

"Next?"

Rule 7

Hug a Patient, Hire a Lawyer

WESTERN MEDICINE IS A strict, hands-off discipline. In our squeaky-clean society, any therapeutic laying on of hands is done with rubber gloves. This is too bad. The caress of a shaman's hand on a fevered body has sometimes cured, always comforted. If a patient sprains her back, I hope she does it in Kyoto where, after a hot bath, she'll get a shiatsu massage. If she sprains it in Chicago, she'll be handed a prescription for a muscle relaxant that can wipe out her bone marrow.

Small wonder American patients line up to put their aching backs in the sturdy hands of chiropractors. In my opinion, chiropractors, hands down, are no more therapeutic than breakfast cereal. Snap. Crackle. Pop.

Those of us in more orthodox medical fields are best advised to keep our hands to ourselves. Hugs, for instance, are highly therapeutic, but a friendly hug around a lonely waist can release erotic energies. Before a doctor knows it, he is paying $40 to lie down in a motel room and $1,000,000 to stand up in a courtroom. As magically as a kiss can transform certain frogs into princes, a hug can change a patient into a plaintiff.

If a malpractice lawyer should ever find out that I'm a Hugging Doctor, he'll be so happy he'll want to hug me.

Rule 8

If You Don't Believe in Prescribing Xanax for Your Anxious Patients, Be Sure to Take One Yourself

---

IN ADDITION TO THEIR physical symptoms, most patients suffer from serious anxiety or depression—at least mine do. If a doctor doesn't think *his* do, then he is using either charm or aloofness to shield himself from his patients.

Nothing irritates me more than a patient's vehement refusal to take Xanax for his anxiety when he doesn't hesitate to knock back six ounces of gin to unwind at night. In the process of unwinding my patient, alcohol damages his brain cells and liver cells. Taken in moderation, Xanax works immoderately well to get my tense patients through their days and nights—and me through mine—with brain and liver cells intact.

Yes, I take Xanax once in a while. After the thirty-fifth phone call and twenty-third patient, I often get tense. If I were organically depressed rather than intermittently anxious, I wouldn't hesitate to take Wellbutrin each morning. I'd be crazy not to.

Mankind has always sought chemical relief from anxiety. Like most people, I've experimented with alcohol, nicotine, and caffeine, often at one sitting. I've seen what these seductive poisons do to me and my patients. I've concluded that if booze, cigarettes, and coffee suddenly became extinct, so would doctors.

Not that tranquilizers and antidepressants are my only defense against patients' emotional upheavals. I'm also in favor of using non-pharmacologic agents, especially meditation, massage, and meatballs in marinara sauce.

Beyond that, I have made a point of learning who are the most compassionate and intuitive psychotherapists in my community—they all happen to be women—and I refer my frazzle-brained and brokenhearted patients to them in droves. I'm convinced that a combination of pharmacotherapy and psychotherapy works better than either alone.

Speaking of drugs, I don't keep morphine or Demerol in my office or my doctor's bag. They tempt the burglar latent in the junkie; they tempt the junkie latent in the doctor.

Rule 9

Kill as Few Patients as Possible

THE OLD MAN SEATED on the end of the examining table removed his perfect smile and wrapped it in a paper towel. I was about to examine his throat with my indirect laryngoscope and had asked him to take out his dentures. I grabbed his tongue with a gauze flat and slid the lighted tube to the back of the pharynx. At that moment the light-bulb dropped off the end of the instrument and lodged in his larynx. Panic-stricken, I jerked out the instrument, let go of his tongue and smacked him sharply on his upper back. The lightbulb shot out of his mouth, flew across the room, and shattered against a wall. "Are you finished, Doc?" he asked, wiping his mouth with the back of his hand.

"Yep, Ed, I'm finished."

That was as close as I've come to killing a patient without his consent. From that day on, I left the laryngoscopic examination of my patients to the otaryngologists and their presumably superior instruments.

Rule 10

Give a Patient Your Best Shot

EVERY NOW AND THEN a doctor will see a patient who has never had a tetanus shot; if the doc is having a bad day, the patient will impart this information through clenched teeth. The doctor is then plunged into the abyss of treating lockjaw, which has a 50 percent mortality. He would, of course, have prevented this disaster if he had injected the patient every ten years with a booster shot of tetanus toxoid.

With a silent prayer, I also give an occasional shot of lidocaine and corticosteroid into an inflamed shoulder or knee joint not responsive to swallowed toxins. (Why ship this patient off to an orthopedic surgeon who will get all the glory and twice my fee for the same injection?) The results of an intra-articular injection are often so spectacular that I have to restrain the patient from asking for another shot too soon. Otherwise I might end up with a waiting room crowded with moon-faced cortisone junkies. These moonies, as it were, become fanatically devoted to their shot-happy doctors.

If you're going to shoot a patient, do it right. A good way to make an enemy for life is to work the needle's tip into the patient's flesh *slowly* in a misguided effort to spare him suffering. Not to put too fine a point on it, you must harpoon your patient with the syringe. Or, rather, with your fingertips hold the syringe like a dart and *toss* it with a snap of the wrist into the bulge of the patient's upper arm. You needn't stand across the room to achieve this effect; sidle up to the patient, get that needle in fast and you will receive one of the sweetest compliments in medicine.

"I didn't feel a thing! You give a good shot, Doc."

"Don't call me 'Doc.'"

One of the most pernicious habits a doctor can develop is injecting vitamin B12 into a patient who complains of fatigue. (*All* patients complain of fatigue.) As any first-year medical student knows, the only disease requiring an injection of B12 (or cyanocobalamin as it's called in medical school) is pernicious anemia, an exceedingly rare malady.

The wealthiest doctor in my town either made his fortune giving unnecessary B12 shots or had cornered the world's entire population of pernicious anemia victims. It is estimated that his Mercedes got over three hundred miles to each gallon of cyanocobalamin. I am sad to report that this dear and glorious quack died in his late seventies of—yes!—pernicious anemia. Like the plague doctor of yore, he was a victim of the very illness he had devoted his career to abolishing. They never taught me in medical school that pernicious anemia could be as contagious as avarice.

Rule 11

Don't Forget to Make a Cameo Appearance at Your Office Daily

So REPELLENT IS THE practice of medicine to some doctors that they will go to any length to avoid putting in an appearance at the office. These doctors are usually married to wealthy spouses and therefore can afford to indulge their aversion to seeing patients. They could, of course, retire from medicine, but a doctor in his thirties who no longer practices medicine invites speculation of drug abuse, sexual misconduct, or perverse golfing practices. To avoid seeing patients, these miscast doctors will accept revolting appointments to hospital committees; they will sign up for conventions in southern climes and spend the prime of their lives sitting sunburned in darkened auditoriums while a fellow goof-off in shorts drones through a microphone about the differential diagnosis of edema.

Were I to make the mistake of looking at the next day's office schedule, I myself would be tempted to run screaming to the nearest airport. So I have learned not to scan my appointment book in advance. I arrive on time each morning at my office and let the horror of the day's appointments unfold gradually. For this exemplary willingness to take what comes, I sometimes reward myself with a three-hour lunch break, making certain to put in a cameo appearance at the office sometime during the afternoon.

Rule 12

Join a Partnership and Die Rich, Young, and Anonymous

In PRIMARY-CARE MEDICINE, solo practice is the only way to fly. Young physicians flock to group practices out of a misguided need for self-protection. They have just emerged pale and shaken from the dark night of their hospital training—years of watching patients die in response to their best efforts. They are under the impression that private practice is more of the same. The thought of facing all that death and dying alone drives them into the many-armed embrace of that false deity, Group Practice. As members of a group, they proceed to blur their identities and work twice as hard as Soloists. Members of a group make a lot of money, lose a lot of friends (their partners), and die young. When news of the death hits the medical community, the departed is eulogized with a poignant, "Who's he?"—or with the more personal remembrance, "Wasn't he with Sol's group?"

As a solo practitioner, I expect to outlive every groupie in town. For one thing, I don't work as hard. A solo doctor is in a better position to say no than a group of doctors. A group always has someone available to take anything that comes over the phone or through the door; they end up swamped. When I get pressed, I have my receptionist say, "I'm sorry, but Dr. London is no longer accepting new patients. Why don't you try calling that new group in town, Drs. Rich, Young, and Anonymous, Inc.?"

To survive in solo practice you, of course, must have a good sign-out schedule. I share night-call, weekends, and vacations with five other solo internists. When I'm away, they take care of my patients just as well, if not better, than the World's Best Doctor.

When I return to work, I'm happy to see my name up there, alone, on the door. The best-kept secrets of private practice are that patients don't die very often during the span of your career and that almost all their illnesses would go away without you. At least 90 percent of my patients are lovely people. Why would I want a group to protect me from all these wonderful folks?

Rule 13

When You Make a Mistake So Horrible It's to Die Over, Don't

My phone rings at 3:04 a.m. It's an emergency-room doctor calling from a small hospital a hundred miles away. It seems that the patient I sent out of my office the previous afternoon with a diagnosis of flu has just died of multiple pulmonary emboli. At 3:04 that morning, some schlepper in the boonies is telling me that he made the diagnosis I missed. I sent the patient home with a smile and a pat on the back—he had traveled a hundred miles to see me, the World's Best Doctor—and now he lies dead from a disease I should have diagnosed while there was time to save him. I thank the emergency room doctor for the information and am told the patient's wife wants to talk to me.

At this point I want to trade places with the patient. What do I do instead?

I tell the wife that I am terribly sorry her husband has died and that I missed the diagnosis completely. When I hang up, I begin my survival training. I smack my forehead once, hard, and acknowledge that I was the World's Biggest Jerk to think the man's profuse sweating and his slight shortness of breath were due to the flu. His lungs sounded fine, his chest film was normal, and I blew the diagnosis to hell and the patient to God knows where.

Within a week, if I haven't died of self-flagellation, I pick up the phone to hear the soft, compassionate voice of a malpractice lawyer wanting to ask me "a few questions" about the case. I refer him to my own lawyer and hang up. I have blundered horribly and no one can make me pay more than the price I exact from myself.

When I have made a catastrophic mistake, I ask myself, How am I going to get out of this one alive? With the clarity of hindsight, I pinpoint where I went wrong with the case. At least if the same situation arises again—it never does—I won't make the same mistake.

For at least two weeks I go around wearing an eighty-pound leaden vest of grief. To get it off my chest, I seek out a confidant or pay for one: a psychotherapist. I stay in shape. I get eight hours of drugged sleep each night. I eat three small meals a day, exercise, and meditate. I keep away from alcohol. I try to stay sharp for the patients I must continue to see.

I don't take "a few days off" or have "just a little drink"—this can add up to a forty-year toot at the end of which the few patients I have left in my office will insist on calling me "Doc."

As a doctor, I must keep myself intact while I wall off the horror of human imperfection. Until the next time.

Rule 14

Honor the Aged

THE MEN AND WOMEN over the age of seventy-five in my practice are my nobility. An eighty-year-old widow insists she feels like the same person she was at twenty-five and asks what she is doing in her grandmother's body; this observation entitles her to the rank of duchess in my book. Her arthritically handknit sweater is composed of 75 percent wool, 15 percent polyester, and 10 percent cat hair, but to my eyes it's pure ermine.

The Duchess and her peers have taught me, a peon of somewhat lesser age, a thing or two. For instance, it takes at least seventy-five years to recover from the five basic mistakes we are all privileged to make if we should live so long. These mistakes embrace our education, our love lives, our careers, our roles as parents, and our investments. I bow to anyone who has been through all that—plus illness and bereavement—and shows up at my office smiling. I bow to anyone who hasn't got long to live.

Last year, the eighty-year-old Duchess suffered a massive stroke that left her unable to speak or comprehend. Her right arm and leg were paralyzed. Half the visual field in each of her eyes was gone. Five days later, she was no better. A neurologist I called in said there was no hope for improvement. She lay in her bed staring half-sighted, half-witted at the ceiling. Whenever her right arm or leg was moved, she groaned in pain.

Long before she suffered this disaster, the Duchess had given me a clear signal to keep her out of a nursing home at all costs. With the unanimous consent of her family, I deprived the nursing home of a patient. How? Simple—she was given no intravenous fluids, and plenty of morphine for her pain. Two days later, with her daughter stroking her forehead, the Duchess quietly died.

Three notes to my own doctor: 1. When I get to be eighty, call me "Duke." 2. Don't call me "Doc." 3. When my time comes, let me die clasped in the arms of Morpheus rather than live strapped to a chair before the Sony in the day room.

Rule 15

Don't Be Late for Your Own Happy Hour

ONE WAY TO SURVIVE the agony of a day in the office is to schedule an hour of escape each night after the last patient leaves. For doctors in paperback novels, this nocturnal diversion becomes a tedious ritual of dry martinis and moist paramours. I myself have found solace at twilight in twenty minutes of meditation, followed by forty of P. G. Wodehouse. "Plum" (as Pelham Grenville's friends called him) was writing at the top of his form in his nineties when he died, presumably laughing.

I'm not sure what I'll take up when I run out of Wodehouse—probably something British again. The United Kingdom, it seems, nurtures the best humorists, gin, and paramours.*

---

*Wodehouse, Waugh, Wilde; Beefeater, Bombay, Boords; E. Ternan, E. Terry, E. Taylor.

Rule 16

Since Death Is Very Still, Keep Moving

I HAVE NEVER WITNESSED a death that hasn't taught me something about how to live. Let me tell you of the deaths of a Jewish butcher and a Catholic widow.

I had never felt such strength in another man. I tried to hold him down in bed by forcing back his shoulders. Up he came, wild-eyed, clutching his chest. He sat for a moment in the center of his deathbed and then lunged for the side rails. We began a fierce bout of arm wrestling as I tried to get him to lie down. I was an intern, age twenty-three, and would live for decades; he was a retired butcher, age seventy-six, and would live for a few seconds. Dying, he was twice as strong as I, living.

"Lie down, Jake," I cried. "I want to give you something for your pain!"

"No, damn you!" he shouted, and fell back dead. All my efforts and those of other young doctors who had come running could not retrieve him from his sudden, profound inactivity.

As I stood over his spent body, my hands and arms still throbbed from his powerful grip. It took weeks for his blue fingerprints to fade from my body. I realized that in his fight to the finish, I had not been his opponent; I had been the referee trying to stop an uneven match.

I have been in physical training ever since. I want to live as long as Jake the butcher and go out as he did—a charging bull.

The corpse of the eighty-three-year-old widow sat staring at her TV set in the living room. By the time I arrived at her house, her family and priest were there. I had little to do but offer my condolences and turn off the TV. The young priest was in a wonderful mood; he had just dispatched another soul to heaven, first-class, nonstop, absolutely and positively. (When it comes to ambience in a house of mourning, give me Catholics every time.)

The priest was smiling as he said, "What do you think she died of, Doc? Boredom?"

"I'm sure of it, Padre," I said. "But on the death certificate, I don't think I can list Lawrence Welk reruns as the immediate cause of death."

We all had a good laugh over that exchange. Even the deceased was grinning.

It took the death of a Catholic widow to teach this Jewish doctor that there is television after life.

Rule 17

Eschew Long White Coats and Polyester Suits

I LIKE TO TELL medical students the story of the dapper salesman in his early seventies who almost choked to death on a forkful of chopped liver at his grandson's bar mitzvah. Of course, what you have an abundance of at any Jewish celebration, besides chopped liver, is physicians. When the stricken salesman fell to his knees, clutching his throat, the doctors in the room ended up taking numbers to see who would be the first in line to perform the Heimlich maneuver. It fell to young Dr. Barry Shapiro to save the patient's life. Not only did Dr. Shapiro perform a successful Heimlich, but in loosening the salesman's collar he discovered a tiny thyroid nodule and a faintly pulsating carotid aneurysm. Even his colleagues on the sidelines were impressed.

When the salesman regained consciousness, he looked up at his young savior and cried, "Get me a doctor!"

"But I *am* a doctor," protested Shapiro, presenting the patient with his card.

"Get outta here," said the salesman. "You're wearing a polyester suit and a floral-print tie and you call yourself a *doctor*?"

Almost as important as avoiding polyester suits and floral-print ties is *not* wearing a long white coat in the office. Long white coats are for Professors of Medicine and your more high-priced television repairmen, the ones who don't make housecalls. Short white jackets are for interns and residents.

As befits the World's Best Doctor, I wear a subdued, but not funereal, suit or sports jacket and a coordinated tie. I don't worry about getting my fine clothes stained by my patients' precious bodily fluids; a damp gauze sponge and a dab of liquid soap work wonders on any spot.

I never fail to brush my shoes and teeth, pausing only to change brushes. On a bad day, a smile and a shoeshine may be the only things I have going for me.

When I neglect to trim my hair and nails, I remind myself that Dr. Jekyll always kept *his* hair and nails trimmed; Mr. Hyde didn't.

Rule 18

Don't Weintraub Yourself to Death

WHEN I WAS A medical student, the class joke was a *kvetch* by the name of Merton Weintraub. With each breath, he drew in panic and exhaled desolation. It was my misfortune to have him quartered upstairs from me in a boardinghouse near the medical school.

If a final exam were scheduled in the morning, Weintraub would sit at his desk a maximum of three minutes and then get up to pace and moan. I could hear the process in high fidelity amplified by the wooden flooring between us. First the scrape of his chair on the bare hardwood, then the doomed, rhythmic squeak of his pacing. Out of his open window and down into mine would drift a high-pitched nasal keening. It was a sound so mournful, the birds in the maple tree outside would grow silent and the faint breeze in the leaves would die.

At this point I would take a broom handle and rap the ceiling three times. The squeaking would stop and the moaning would drop an octave in pitch. Worse yet, often as not, I would then hear his leaden footsteps coming down the spiral staircase.

To my study-strained eyes, he looked like the last survivor of Custer's party at Little Big Horn; it appeared he had been scalped and five arrows protruded from his chest. But no, Weintraub was simply a victim of premature baldness and never ventured forth without five ballpoint pens bristling in his shirt pocket.

"I can't study," he would announce.

"For Christ's sake, Weintraub," I said, "stop worrying. The worst that can happen to you is you'll flunk the test, get kicked out of medical school, and be returned to your parents on a blue shield."

"Thanks, I knew you'd understand," he said, shuffling out of my room and slamming the door behind him. For a few moments I listened to the robins in the maple tree and savored the lilac-scented breeze wafting through my window. And then, the scraping, the squeaking, and the moaning.

Weintraub invested no less agony in choosing a weekend date, deciding between soup and salad on a menu, or in pondering the causes of the fleeting chest pains he was prone to.

He got through medical school, graduating summa cum laude over my almost-dead body downstairs.

His next problem was trying to decide which of seven internships he should accept. It was the last night we would spend under the same roof, and Weintraub's pacing and moaning kept me awake until 2 A.M. Against my better judgment, I grabbed the broomstick and gave the ceiling three good ones, knocking loose some plaster. The pacing and moaning continued unabated for a few moments. A short silence ensued, following by a house-shaking thud.

I managed to resuscitate him before the ambulance arrived, but he died the next day in the university hospital. He barely made the deadline for the medical school yearbook, becoming the first obituary of the class of '55. The pressured typesetter misspelled his name, *Wientraub*. Had Weintraub lived to see this typo, I think it would have killed him.

When I attended the twenty-fifth reunion of our graduating class, I made the mistake of taking my old room in the boardinghouse for the night. At three in the morning, I was startled awake by the sound of chair legs scraping above me. A rhythmic squeak followed, then a familiar nasal keening. Every two minutes I could hear the distant lament, "Not *Wien*traub, you dyslexic dipshit, WEINtraub."

Since then, if I catch myself Weintraubing, I pour three ounces of Bombay gin over ice and put a Schubert sonata on my CD player.

Rule 19

Feed a Cold, Starve a Lawyer

WHENEVER I PRESCRIBE AN antibiotic drug for, say, a strep throat, I admonish the patient, "Eat well, rest well, get well." My mother taught me this excellent holistic advice during the course of my premedical training, otherwise known as a Jewish childhood. An orthodox therapist, she replaced the precious bodily fluids I lost through fever with those of a chicken, lost through boiling.

Which came first, the chicken or the aspirin, is a question that is beyond the scope of this treatise.

If, indeed, we are what we eat, then I am mostly bull, a little chicken, something of a pig, and hardly a cold fish. Whenever I find myself standing in line before a magnificent buffet table, I never fail to acknowledge my gratitude for the place I've been assigned in the biologic food chain.

I am about fifteen pounds overweight by most standard tables (kitchen, dining room, and buffet) and therefore cut a poor figure as a role model for proper nutrition. In my secret heart, I believe a deeply enjoyed meal in a three-star restaurant can add six months to your life. If I'm wrong, I can think of no better time to die than between the Grand Marnier soufflé and the presentation of the bill at Taillevent in Paris. Just wheel me out on the dessert cart to the black Citroën limo in the alley.

To those who seek immortality on the shelves of health food stores, I say, "He who eats groats, bloats." I suppose the controlled emission of all that gas can facilitate jogging. (*Tail wind*, I think, is the technical term runners use.) Without putting too fine a point on it, I'd rather be carted out at sixty then farted out at ninety.

Dr. London's Save-Your-Life Diet

Breakfast

Poached egg, half-slice dry toast, 2 ounces orange juice

Lunch

1 ounce boiled tofu, 8 ounces ice water

Dinner

3 ounces fresh beluga caviar

4 ounces goose-liver pâté with port jelly

Lobster bisque

Puff pastry stuffed with boned woodchuck and truffles

Châteaubriand grilled medium rare over mesquite charcoal;
sauce Béarnaise

Potatoes lyonnaise

White asparagus tips sautéed in sweet butter

Green salad tossed with extra-virgin olive oil and balsamic
vinegar, overlaid with a trellis of 7 medium anchovy fillets

Assorted cheeses, fruit

Coffee (NO CREAM)

Chocolates (Bonbonniér de Palace, Lausanne)

Champagne (Schramsberg Cuvée de Pinot), throughout

Rule 20

Execute Insurance Forms at Dawn

INSURANCE FORMS ARE THE cockroaches of a medical office and should be dispatched at once, before they take over the premises. If allowed to multiply, insurance forms (and their prolific cousins, disability forms and work-injury forms) can sorely tempt the physician to commit arson or suicide.

I have a family in my practice whose members have lifted themselves out of poverty and plunged me into depression by mastering the art of self-inflicted personal injury in public places. The combined efforts of the Bustamontes have generated the nastiest forms I've ever wept over. Their modus operandi is to slip on fallen fruit in supermarkets, trip over footstools in shoe stores, fall into holes dug by sewer districts, step in front of small foreign cars moving slowly through intersections, climb over hospital bed side-rails and dive headfirst for the floor. On a quiet afternoon, I can stand on any downtown street corner and hear the distant thud of a Bustamonte. In homage to the Flying Wallendas, I have named them the Diving Bustamontes. I have often thought of resigning from their care, but I haven't the heart to inflict the Bustamontes or their forms on a beloved colleague—or even a hated one. The only way I can keep pace is to examine the stricken Bustamonte in a hurry and fill out the form before he or she can fall off my examining table.

Rule 21

Don't Hang Mirrors in Your Waiting Room
Unless Your Two O'Clock Patient Enjoys
Watching Himself Age Visibly by Four P.M.

I AM FOND OF telling patients whom I've kept waiting for more than sixty minutes, "About twenty years ago, I got two hours behind and I haven't quite caught up yet." My patients, somehow, are not as fond of this story as I am.

After the first patient of the day, I am never on time. The scheduled chaos of private practice makes me a little late; the unscheduled chaos makes me very late. I am not happy about this, but neither am I stricken with guilt. The people out there flipping through old *New Yorkers* are waiting for medical care, not public transportation. The Streetcar Named Disease is never on schedule and has but one destination—the End of the Line. Be patient, patient.

Every now and then one of my patients correctly thinks his or her time is at least as valuable as mine and quits my practice in a huff. "Good for him or her!" I say. "Good riddance!" I add.

Let this affronted clockwatcher find a doctor who is always on time and the two of them can race each other to the morgue.

"Next?"

Rule 22

Don't Call a Rose a Rose; Call Her Mrs. Schwartz

I ONCE CAUGHT A former receptionist of mine addressing an elderly patient who had just come to the window, "Hi, Rose. Have a seat. Dr. London will see you in a few minutes."

Outraged, the patient, a jaundiced dowager from Dallas, said, "How *dare* you call me 'Rose'! Tell *Oscar* that *Mrs. Schwartz* has decided to find another doctor."

I immediately dashed into the waiting room to apologize. It was no go. The Yellow Rose of Texas—as I came to call her—was lost and gone forever. "Dreadful sorry, Clementine," I said to my receptionist, "you're fired. You should never call patients by their first names unless they ask you to."

"Drop dead, Oscar," she replied.

To this day, I find myself having to stifle an impulse to call patients, especially young ones, by their first names. Medical etiquette, as I see it, demands that the doctor offer to let Mrs. Rose Schwartz call him by *his* first name if he wants to address Mrs. Schwartz by *her* first name. To the receptionist, a Rose by any other name is still Mrs. Schwartz, until further notice.

As a result of adhering to his principle, I am Oscar to a dozen Roses and Dr. London to an equal number of Mrs. Schwartzes. I rather like this mixture—I don't want a room full of Roses.

Rule 23

Keep Banker's Hours

I'm in my office weekdays only from ten to twelve and two to five. Like every mother's son the golfer, I take Wednesday afternoons off. This somewhat less than back-breaking schedule gives me enough time each morning to meditate for twenty minutes, exercycle for thirty minutes, and read for an hour. At noon I can spend two hours on a languid lunch or a serious nap. With my last appointment at 4:30 in the afternoon, I am able to get home at night well before 1 a.m.

My banker's hours permit me to make the odd housecall in the morning, or the even odder dash to the emergency room over the lunch hour, without seriously jamming my schedule. If an inordinate number of patients call in acutely ill, I have the extra time to work them in without becoming a patient myself. My banker's hours allow me to make slightly more than a cameo appearance in my office.

Traditionally, I spend my Wednesday afternoons at the golf course, lurking behind bushes and shooting my colleagues in their buttocks with a BB gun. I like to get them as they are bending down to mark their balls on the greens. Keeps them on their toes. This pastime may seem odd to you, but I've always thought it important for a doctor to cultivate an eccentricity; otherwise he runs the risk of being stereotyped. So, I shoot doctors on golf courses.

There's something about that endless expanse of grass, the lovely trees, the flapping flag at every hole, and the sherbet-colored slacks of my colleagues at play that excites the sporting instinct in me. I'm not very good, actually. On my best afternoon I shot only a sixty-four: seventeen internists, eight ophthalmologists, fourteen general surgeons, nineteen family practitioners and—on the back nine—six proctologists and a partridge in a pear tree. (The last quite by accident, I assure you.)

If you think my golfing story puts too much stress on your suspension of disbelief, just ask any doctor in my town which of his colleagues is the biggest pain in the ass.

Rule 24

Don't Plant Time Bombs in Your Office

I MAY ALWAYS BE LATE, but I never waste time. Like a blackjack pro counting cards, I watch every move my patients make. I can look at a patient's fingernails for one second and make the diagnosis of chronic arsenic poisoning that another doctor missed during thirty half-hour visits over five years. If I lose my concentration, then *I* become the schlemiel some hotshot internist one-ups five years later.

In my practice, I've got to move fast but not so fast that I empty my office of problems that come back to haunt me. I don't want to send a malignant melanoma out my door because I'm too rushed to have my patient fully disrobe during a checkup. That melanoma is a time bomb that will explode two years later when I finally detect it—far advanced—on the back of my patient's thigh. If I had taken a few moments to check the patient's skin two years before, he would now be cured instead of imminently dead.

I have to be ruthless with my time. I can effectively deal with the sore throat of an established patient in three minutes. Then I have twenty-five minutes to examine, at some leisure, a new patient with chronic back pain who has brought in a thirty-five-pound stack of old X-rays. I know at a glance that his back pain is caused by hauling that load of films to countless consultants, but I'll need twenty-five minutes to get up the courage to tell him.

Rule 25

Make a Housecall and Become a Legend in Your Own Time

IF THE PATIENT CAN withstand the shock, I offer to make a housecall. Once I get there, I never regret it. A housecall is such a novelty these days that the patient's family can't do enough to express their gratitude.

"You're a saint to come all the way out here to see Grandpa!"

"Can I take your coat?"

"Would you like a cup of coffee?"

"How about a sixty-four piece set of sterling silver? Sheldon, carry the silver to the doctor's car."

Of course, if the *patient* had received this much loving care from his family, he wouldn't have needed a housecall in the first place.

The fact remains that sometimes a patient is too sick to get out of bed to see the doctor. Rather than punish him for his infirmity by having an ambulance drag race him to the nearest emergency room, the doctor can jolly well hitch up the horse and buggy and go out in the snowstorm to the patient's bedside. Although the horse and buggy have been replaced by the four-wheel drive, the only modern way to cope with a snowstorm is to practice in Palm Springs.

Despite the time and trouble, I have almost always found the housecall a vivid experience. Last year I paid a visit to the bedside of a dying cellist. The elderly veteran of the symphony lay propped up on one half of a double bed, staring straight ahead. His cancer of the liver had spread widely since my last visit. His thin, jaundiced body with its distended abdomen was a grotesque caricature of the very instrument he played. His silver-haired wife was a blur of activity in contrast to his stillness. She took my coat, plumped up his pillows, pulled over a chair for me, and turned on the bedside lamp.

After I examined the patient, I was hard put to say anything that would comfort him or his wife. I followed his gaze and noticed his gorgeous cello—as silent and delicate as the patient—standing against the wall. The old, deeply polished instrument lay inside a new padded vinyl case that stood open.

"I bought Herman a new case for his cello, just before he got sick," said his wife, her eyes brimming.

My God, I thought, he's staring at his own funeral!

"The cello and the case are beautiful," I said, looking up at the wife. "But let me suggest you carry them out to the hall."

With a slightly hurt look, she obeyed. While she was out of the room, the patient's face relaxed. He smiled at me and said, "Thank you, doctor. I didn't want to hurt Gerda's feelings."

When she returned to the room, the patient had drifted into the first peaceful sleep he had had in days. He never woke up.

Rule 26

Don't Try to Feel a Breast Lump Over the Telephone

THE MOMENT A WOMAN calls to say she's discovered a breast lump, I tell her to come over at once. Until I see her, she's in a frenzy of suspense.

I usher her into the exam room as soon as she arrives—no *New Yorkers* for her. If the lump feels suspicious, I explain right off that I'd like to have a surgeon biopsy it. She's expecting the worst anyway, so there's no use telling her, "Don't worry—there's always a chance it's benign" or "Don't worry—let's get mammograms" or "Don't worry—lots of lumps go away by themselves, blah, blah, blah." Get her to the best surgeon in town, who will cut out the blah, blah, blah —and the lump.

When she goes into the hospital, I visit her every day and don't, for God's sake, charge her. (This book is not subtitled How to Be the World *Richest* Doctor.) If the lump is benign, I celebrate with her; if it's malignant, I tell her every happy story I know about twenty-year survivals. Indeed, I've stuck around long enough to have patients thank me twenty years after their mastectomies just for having been there.

Rule 27

Never Let a Patient Outflank You

WHAT I'M ABOUT TO relate happened to me only once, because I've not allowed it to happen to me again.

Mr. Axel Boone was a forty-seven-year-old, sunburned steve-dore who was seeing me for the first time. Powerfully muscled, soft-spoken, and vaguely menacing, he sat stripped to the waist on the exam table. His massive torso and arms reminded me of the lower third of a redwood trunk and its first two limbs. I asked him what was troubling him and he growled, "I hurt my back at work."

Oh God—a work-injury case! The endless forms! The lingering symptoms!

I had agreed to see Mr. Boone at the behest of his wife who had been a gracious and blissfully uncomplaining patient of mine for years. And now here was her Axel claiming to have been injured while lifting a crate on a loading dock. I can't resist pointing out that I myself felt like a doc on whom a crate had just been unloaded.

"Is it your lower back or your upper back that hurts?" I asked.

"Both," he offered, challengingly.

It was at this point that I made my strategic blunder. I turned my back to the patient and began scribbling a note on his chart on the countertop. Suddenly I felt a blunt object prodding my back between my shoulder blades. My blood froze. Instinctively, I began to raise my arms over my head.

"Here's where it hurts, Doc," said Mr. Boone. "Then it travels up here."

To my vast relief, he was slowly tracing the anatomical map of his pain—on my back—with his index finger. I was out of danger, but far from comfortable.

Having finished writing my note, I would by this time have turned to face him again, but he had me pinned. For an eternal minute and a half he laboriously sketched the migrations of his pain between my scapulae, up to my cervical spine, across my right rib cage, and down to my fifth lumbar vertebra.

By nature I am ticklish, but by training I try not to laugh out loud in the presence of a patient—especially a 230-pound stevedore. By the time he had completed his pointed, nonverbal description of his symptoms, I was tied up in knots from my head to my pelvis and was about to pop from repressed hilarity.

More important, the World's Best Doctor had made an accurate diagnosis with his back turned to the patient. It was an open-and-shut case of Malingering. No genuine pain suffered by man or beast ever traveled a more circuitous and neurologically meaningless route as did Mr. Boone's alleged backache.

Unskewered at last, I wheeled around and said, "That's *some* pain you have, Mr. Boone."

"You better believe it."

It was now *my* turn to go over *his* back. Whereas his pointed digit tickled, my gently probing fingers elicited groans of the most excruciating pain.

"You're killing me, Doc."

"You slay me, Mr. Boone."

We had just exchanged back-to-back accusations of murder. I chose not to request that he refrain from calling me "Doc."

Rather than confront him with my diagnosis on his first visit, I suggested that we get the obligatory X-rays and reconvene in my office the following week.

"Hey, Doc," he said, as I started to walk out of the examining room, "I also got this pulled groin muscle."

He made a move toward me, but I was face-to-face this time with my adversary. I protectively covered myself with his chart and backed out of the room.

After his X-rays came back negative the following Thursday, I turned the case over to Mrs. Boone, who had him back on the job the next day.

Rule 28

Praise Nurses and Your Patients Will Live Forever or Die Happy

WORKING WITH A GOOD nurse is one of the great joys of being a doctor. I cannot understand physicians who adopt a hostile relationship with nurses. They are depriving themselves of an education in hospital wisdom and are robbing their patients of round-the-clock loving care. A nurse who's miffed at a doctor can hardly be blamed for a certain coolness toward his patients—unless the nurse is a saint, as not a few are.

When I was a young doctor starting out in practice, I wasn't about to let a crusty RN tell this newborn MD how to practice medicine. Only after some years did I discover that a good nurse, like a good loaf of bread, is the staff of life, and the crustier the better.

Nurses have taught me to pull aside the bedsheet so that the lower half of a patient's body does not become a stamping ground for malpractice lawyers. (Decubitus ulcers, thrombophlebitis, perianal abscesses, and gangrenous toes are among the snappy tunes lawyers love to dance to.) A good coronary care nurse is one of the best cardiologists I'll ever meet. When the nurse suggests stopping the quinidine, I stop the quinidine.

Nurses have taught me the intensive care that only compassion provides. Compassion is the conspiracy a good nurse forms with a patient to combat the inhumanity of hospitalization. ("When you get back from your barium enema, Mrs. Glick, I'll have your lunch and a back rub waiting for you.")

I've had a nurse walk up to me and say the patient I admitted with "fever of unknown origin" had been bitten by a tick in Colorado the week before and was now probably in the early stages of Rocky Mountain spotted fever. Damned if she wasn't right. And what did the World's Best Doctor do after he wiped the egg off his face? He called up the nursing supervisor and praised the diagnostic acumen of that brilliant nurse to the skies. And when that nurse threw a white angora wrap over her shoulders at 11 P.M., she flashed me the most wickedly triumphant and grateful smile I've ever seen on the face of an angel about to soar up into the night sky.

Rule 29

Don't Be the Last Doc on the Block to Own a Plastic Gallbladder; See a Detail Rep

I'M A PUSHOVER FOR pharmacological salespeople. I've tried to analyze why I allow myself to be propagandized by these well-groomed supplicants of the Corporate Drug Structure. Is it because my father was a struggling shirt salesman? Do I invite a detail rep into my office to keep a drug pusher off the streets? Am I so intellectually starved that my mind hungers for the advertising pap of the caplet cartels? Am I trying to amass the world's largest collection of antihistamine samples? Am I afraid to say no?

None of the above. The reason I see detail reps is their beautiful gifts. I refer to the one-fourth scale, three-dimensional plastic colon—so glistening, pink, and upright on its fragile stand! Through a window in its splenic flexure one can see the lurid red and yellowness of amebic dysentery. My plastic colon makes a perfect centerpiece for our dining room table when we entertain guests who profess to be on diets.

And how I treasure my dozen hollow plastic kidneys! They make ideal bathtub toys for doctors and their children. You've never heard of floating kidneys?

Thanks to the munificence of detail reps, I have a different ball-point pen for every day of the year. I could retire from medicine tomorrow and live for a decade on the sales of my promotional pens, flashlights, tranquilizers, and plastic viscera. ("Good morning, I'm 'Doc' London. Please accept this complimentary Xanax tablet. Can I interest you in a plastic pancreas today?)

The days when drug reps were invariably male are long past. The first day a female detail rep handed a doctor a ballpoint pen was no less auspicious than the day Prosciutto married into the Melon family.

So I am now in the some-would-say enviable position of having intelligent, well-dressed women dying to shower me with gifts. How I love to sit down and listen to them rhapsodize about the half-life of their latest tranquilizer. How I love to fantasize about leaning over my desk and asking one of them if she'd be willing to spend a half-life of tranquility with a middle-aged internist. I can imagine her look of genuine outrage—which would certainly be an improvement on her ersatz gallbladder.

Rule 30

Take Up a Hobby and Become a Multifaceted Bore Instead of a Simple One

AT THE TURN OF the century Sir William Osler, the Best Internist in the Solar System, urged his students to practice medicine as humanitarians, scientists, and artists. In their spare time, he advised, they should take up a hobby. Sir William, that charismatic overachiever, has driven many a lesser physician to an early grave in an effort to emulate him. Here was a Victorian giant who wrote the definitive medical textbook of his age, who was the number-one physician and teacher wherever he settled (Canada, the United States, and England), who had diseases he defined *named* after him—prescribing recreational therapy for us schleppers who are still on the phone with a character disorder at 8 P.M. With all due respect to Sir William, I submit that the only rewarding hobby a modern physician can take up is sleep.

I collect odd hours of sleep like a numismatist collects Indian-head nickels. My most treasured sleep takes place during the twenty minutes that follow the departure of my last patient. I sit alone in my consultation room and recite my mantra three times ("Osler, Os-ler, O-o-ss-ler") and fall into a dreamless sleep. I awake rejuvenated and for a few moments contemplate the joys of not having taken up a conventional hobby.

Instead of standing navel-deep in muck waiting to kill a duck, I gently swivel my hips in the wide-bodied comfort of my office chair and gaze at a painting of an English garden—a fireworks display of rhododendrons in full bloom. I'd rather contemplate a garden than cultivate one. All that mulching of rank, decomposed matter to bring forth sweet-scented, multihued life has terrific spiritual appeal but is very hard on the back.

I am of the W. C. Fields school of gardening. Friends report that he stood on the balcony of his Hollywood estate dressed in naught but a terrycloth bathrobe and surveyed his rose bushes down below with a telescope. After a few minutes of exhausting perusal, he turned to a blackboard and scrawled in chalk, "Bloom you bastards!" As a gardener, W. C. Fields had a red nose instead of a green thumb. He remains an inspiration to us dedicated nonhobbyists.

I cannot end this disquisition on the physician as hobbyist without a few words on photography. Show me a physician with a digital camera around his neck and I will show you a menace to polite society. He comes home from Europe with two thousand photos, of which he deletes seven as being below his standards. He has his wife invite twelve unsuspecting guests for dinner. After dessert, he announces, "Would anyone care to see my photos of Rome, Florence, and Venice? I can hook my computer up to the fifty-nine-inch TV in only a minute."

The guests scan the doors and windows; they are locked; there's no escape. Four hours later the ambulances begin to arrive. The comatose guests are rushed to the nearest emergency room, where huge doses of adrenalin are injected and a pasta-free diet prescribed for one month.

I know a urologist who had the effrontery to conclude a two-hour meal of pot roast, gravy, potatoes, and wine by saying, "I have a few photos of Croatia I'd like to show you."

Halfway through the presentation, a somewhat portly internist rose through a Burgundy stupor and stood before the screen. Lit by an overexposed harbor view, the internist drew a .38-caliber revolver (one of the few weapons more lethal than an 8.3-megapixel camera) and aimed it at the photographer.

"Open the front door, Seymour, and let us out!" shouted the internist. "If you say the word *Dubrovnik* one more time, you're a dead man."

Good night, Sir William, wherever you are.

Rule 31

Review the World Literature Fortnightly

I AM BLESSED WITH a photographic memory. I can read two thousand words a minute and recite them back to you. I subscribe to twenty-seven medical journals, foreign and domestic. I attend over a hundred medical lectures a year. I am lying.

I have based my continuing medical education on the *New England Journal of Medicine*, *The Medical Letter*, and the tape cassettes of *Audio-Digest of Internal Medicine*. I am telling the truth.

The more patients a doctor sees, the fewer journals he has time to read. If he isn't careful, he can end up after forty years with a wealth of experience and a poverty of intellect.

I read the *NEJM* obsessively and listen to *Audio-Digest* tapes religiously. In medical school I was a bookworm; in private practice I'm a tapeworm. I read other journals sporadically and listen to other lectures somnolently.

About once every four years I attend a comprehensive lecture series on internal medicine and catch up on my sleep. Nothing is more conducive to profound sleep than an after-lunch medical lecture given in a hotel ballroom. The lights are dim. The audience is a tranquil sea of slack-jawed men and women in dark-gray and dark-brown suits. Blood is being massively shunted from brains to intestines. Hundreds of eyeballs begin a slow roll upward as the speaker recites the only statement the audience will remember: "May I have the first slide, please?"

I vastly prefer the privacy of my automobile to the lecture hall. As an acoustic shell, the interior of my Lexus rivals Carnegie Hall. What is more, the amenities of Carnegie Hall do not include bucket seats and a sunroof. I drive to and from work with either Mozart soaring or medicine droning. After listening to scores of *Audio-Digest of Internal Medicine* tapes, I have yet to fall asleep at the wheel. The producers of the tapes have a responsibility to keep us awake. An effective way to reduce the population of internists in the country would be to insert the words, "May I have the first slide, please?" into, say, a tape of rheumatoid spondylitis. Perish the thought!

My other source of current medical wisdom is my colleagues' brains. I suck them dry. Mongoose-like, I am forever extracting information from eggheads in the various branches of medicine. I've seen cardiologists cross the street to avoid confronting me. When I've reduced a bright colleague to decerebrate rigidity with my endless questions, he teeters off stiff-legged, thinking he has finally made his escape. But in my best Columbo-Peter Falk imitation, with an upraised arm and finger, I call out, "Uh, one more thing. . . ."

Of course, if a colleague comes up to *me*, the World's Best Doctor, and asks me a medical question, I stare off into the distance and say, "I really don't know. Why don't you look it up online? And let me know what you find out, would you?"

Among my peers, I am admired for my intellectual honesty.

Rule 32

Remember the Brain

I WORRY A LOT about my patients' brains. As Western philosophers point out, "The brain is, you know, where it's at." (At least some *far* Western philosophers put it that way.) For my money, the fundamental goal of a primary-care physician is to save the brain. Whether the patient is a motorcyclist who scoffs at wearing a helmet, a poker player high on drugs and alcohol, or a hypertensive who forgets to take his medication, or—almost as bad—a hypertensive who *remembers* to take his medication, I worry about the brain. (Ernest Hemingway, not one of my patients, went into suicidal depression while he was on reserpine.)

Speaking of brains, I'm reminded of my tour of duty in the Army Medical Corps on Okinawa, where I was in charge of the infectious disease ward. A young marine with fever, headache, and a stiff neck was brought in during the height of an outbreak of Japanese B encephalitis. (In 1958, fortunately, this strain of virus was the only enemy that Americans were fighting in the Pacific.) I had already admitted two dozen patients with this ghastly disease and stood by helplessly as they changed from bright young men to babbling idiots in the time it took them to undress. Many went directly from babble into coma and death.

By the time the young marine with fever, headache, and a stiff neck came under my care I was a hardened veteran of Japanese B encephalitis. I performed a spinal tap on him; as expected, the fluid was clear and grew no bacteria on culture.

Days passed and the ward continued to fill with encephalitis victims, but this one marine stood out from all the rest. First of all, he had the worst headache of the bunch. Second, he was almost fully alert compared to his buddies who were either demented or comatose. After several days, his headache became so intense that thirty milligrams of morphine didn't touch it. He was screaming in pain.

I had read somewhere that a spinal tap itself can sometimes ease the headache of encephalomeningitis. Accordingly, I once again inserted my needle into his spinal cord and out came what looked like coconut milk. Instantly, the patient's headache disappeared; mine had begun.

Under the microscope, the cloudy spinal fluid showed unmistakable evidence of a *bacterial* meningitis. My first tap of his spinal fluid had been too early in his illness to show anything!

I immediately put the patient on sulfa, and he made a full recovery. I can date my worry over my patients' brains from my time on Okinawa when a meningococcus, camouflaged as a virus, stole into camp and almost killed one of my marines.

Rule 33

Don't Let a Shrink Take Credit for Giving Your Patient Prozac

I HAVE NO TROUBLE spotting depressed patients—they're the ones who make *me* depressed. They are the black holes in the cosmos of private practice: people who, given half a chance—or worse, half an hour—will suck you into the void at the center of their being. This is a void from which nothing can escape—not their family, their friends, their doctor, not light itself. When I spot a black hole in my waiting room, I reach for my prescription pad in the shoulder holster of my breast pocket. When the patient sits down and sighs rather than simply inhaling, I brace myself against the gravitational pull and reach for my pen.

In the time it takes this patient to say, "Why am I so tired all the time?" I have written a prescription for Prozac. I make every effort to explain that sometimes the brain can no longer make the biochemicals needed to cope with life's stresses. I invoke a comparison with a diabetic whose pancreas can no longer make insulin. I insist that he or she continue talking to a psychiatrist while starting to take the antidepressant. I cite scores of patients whose ten-year depressions vanished after four weeks on Prozac.

I've learned all I can about Zoloft and Paxil as well as Wellbutrin, MAO inhibitors, and lithium. (I know enough about lithium to let someone else prescribe it.) I've also learned the criteria for electroshock therapy, and if all else fails, I recommend that a mute, motionless patient suffering organic depression be given EST. I have seen dramatic changes for the better: after about the seventh treatment, the black hole implodes and a shining radiance takes its place.

A psychiatrist can work wonders in crisis intervention and grief counseling. But when it comes to organic depression, a shrink, or any other doc, is only as good as the antidepressant the patient is taking.

Rule 34

Let No One Leave Your Office without a Handshake, a Blood Count, and a Smile

---

GOD, DID HE HATE seeing a doctor! A former naval commander, he required a task force of his wife and three daughters to tow him to the office. Since he was too hoarse to speak, his wife explained that he had been having this cold for a week and it was not responding to standard doses of chicken soup and aspirin.

"Now hear this," I said, after examining him and finding nothing except his hoarseness. "The commander will probably sound like a foghorn for three more days until he comes out from under the weather. In the meantime, so his visit here shouldn't be a total loss, I'd like to get a throat culture and draw some blood for a red and white count."

The commander didn't gag when I swabbed his throat nor wince when I drew his blood. Small wonder we won the war in the Pacific!

I gave the commander my best smile and handshake to make up for swabbing his fiery throat and needling his defenseless forearm. Feeling much worse for having seen a doctor, he steamed out of my office at full throttle. He turned once to fire a warning cough at his trailing wife and daughters. They already knew they'd have hell to pay when they reached home port.

The commander's white count was all right. It was his red count that gave me pause. A hemoglobin of 13.2 was much lower than I had expected in this red-blooded American male. I called the commander's wife and instructed her to make an appointment for her husband to get a proctoscopy, a barium enema, and an upper GI series.

The wife left the phone for a few minutes and returned to report that the outraged commander had semaphored that he just had a sore throat for Crissakes and what did he need a goddam ream job for?

After much sound and fury and barium, the commander was found to have a resectable carcinoma of his ascending colon. As they wheeled his gurney down to the operating room, he was shaking his head at the folly of letting his wife and three daughters take him to a doctor for a simple sore throat. Now, twelve years later, he still shakes his head whenever he sees me.

Rule 35

Don't Take Too Much Joy in the Mistakes of Other Doctors

A PATIENT LEAVES ANOTHER practice in high dudgeon and consults me. When she tells me her medical horror story, I'm often tempted to ridicule the jilted doctor. Kicking a colleague when he's down ranks with hitting a Dunlop off a tee as a major medical pastime. Let us say the other doctor prescribed an excessive dose of a sedative, causing the patient to injure herself in an auto accident. How could that meshuggener prescribe two milligrams of Xanax four times a day to this alcoholic woman? What an (*ha-ha!*) outrage! What a (*hee-hee!*) boo-boo! What a (*ho-ho!*) lawsuit!

I make sure the patient lets the other doctor know in writing why she is leaving him. When she disparages him to me, I become uncharacteristically silent. I listen to her lament with great interest and when she simmers down, I say "It sounds like you're terribly unhappy with him." I don't say, "What an outrage! What a boo-boo! What a lawsuit!" If the patient wants legal advice, she has come to the wrong office. Unless the other doctor is a congenital incompetent, I assume he's made one of the ten human errors each physician is cursed with every year. He's probably unhappy enough at losing the patient under these circumstances. Why should I compound his misery by inviting, with an ill-chosen remark, a malpractice lawyer to put in *his* two cents (in hopes of a million-dollar return on his investment)?

I myself came within a whisker of being sued once. A patient of mine happened to have his blood pressure taken by an ophthalmologist in another town. When the eye doctor removed the cuff, he exclaimed, "Who the hell is treating your blood pressure? It's sky-high!"

A malpractice lawyer phoned me a week later. Apologizing for interrupting my busy schedule, he proceeded to regale me with the story of my patient's high blood pressure in the eye doctor's office. When he paused to smack his lips, it's a good thing no one took *my* blood pressure.

I hung up on the lawyer and promptly called the out-of-town ophthalmologist, collect. I sent *his* blood pressure off the top of the gauge with a ten-minute discourse, in words of four and twelve letters, on my learned opinion of a doctor who specializes in the eye and runs off at the mouth.

Rule 36

Don't Use Your Patient as Your Therapist

AMONG THE FEW MEDICAL sins I have not yet committed is using a patient's shoulder to cry on. I've heard about this phenomenon from any number of former patients of other doctors. Internists and psychiatrists seem uniquely disposed to treat suffering patients to several choruses of "You think *you've* got problems!"

The doctor in question can hardly wait for the patient to finish her litany of complaints about say, her rotten marriage, before he pipes up, "The hardest thing in the world is keeping a long marriage viable . . . I should know, I've been tied to the old ball-and-chain for twenty-three years and let me tell you, it's a drag."

Before she knows it, the aggrieved patient is consoling the doctor, pointing out the mitigating delights of domesticity. By the time the visit is over, the doctor feels terrific—ready to take his scuffed ball and rusty chain in for a 10,000-mile checkup—while the patient is left with her rotten husband and a bill for $250. Many a patient cursed with a therapeutic personality has found herself pulling a doctor through his midlife crisis:

Doctor: What can I do for you?
Patient: My knee has started collapsing on me at the oddest times.

Doctor: God, do I sympathize with you! I've had a trick knee myself since college.

Patient: You don't say?

Doctor: Yeah, a football injury in my sophomore year. Torn cartilage. This damn knee (*slaps his right knee*) kept me from playing in the Rose Bowl of '51. (*His eyes mist over.*)

Patient: Gee, Doc, that must have been a blow.

Doctor: Please, don't call me "Doc." Ah well, my bum knee's probably the best thing that ever happened to me. (*Grabs a tissue and blows his nose cathartically.*) While I was laid up after my knee surgery, I really hit the books. This crazy knee (*pats knee affectionately*) probably got me into medical school. And now here I am, ready to help you. What did you say your problem was?

Some doctors—and all dentists—use their patients as captive audiences for their political rantings, their philosophical musings, even their cinematic reviewings. At least the dentist is *working* on the patient while he's dumping on her.

I'm not opposed to all extramedical banter—just the kind that is too self-serving. Once in a while I have to remind myself: it's the patient's visit, not mine.

I admit that at times it's tempting, while bent over a seated Earth Mother with my stethoscope, to drop my weary head on her soft shoulder and blubber, "God, what a day I've had!" A sign to be hung in every examining room: DANGER! SOFT SHOULDER.

Rule 37

When Holes Appear In Your Appointment Schedule, Celebrate

AFTER MORE THAN TWENTY years of active practice I still begin some days with little to do but wonder where it went wrong. It is a Friday, usually the busiest day of the week. Where are the patients? In sheer numbers, the list of names on my day sheet resembles the starting lineup of the local high school basketball team.

Do I worry? Do I fret over a mass defection of my patients? Was it something I said? Or ate? (Too much garlic in the mu-shu pork at the Jaded Palate last night?) Do I, an established internist at the height of his powers, really care if I'm not booked solid? Do I look out the window to see if Dr. Shapiro in the office across the street is listening to a patient's chest with his gold-plated stethoscope?

I used to. And all I'd see was Dr. Shapiro standing at his window looking over at my office to see if I was busy. Feebly, we would wave to one another and go back to staring at our appointment books.

Now when holes appear in my schedule, I rejoice. I use the extra time to linger over the few patients who were good enough to show up; they love it, and so do I. An anemic schedule gives me precious time to complete secondary but important tasks. Time to clip and file my fingernails and medical journals. Time to sort out my drug samples and flush them down the toilet. (When the plumbing in my office goes on the fritz, I don't call a plumber, I call a toxicologist.)

If a hiatus in my schedule occurs after a heavy lunch, I stretch out on an exam table, gaze up at my mobile of paper swallows, and grab forty winks. It is sleep that knits the raveled sleeve of primary care.

When I first began practice, my appointment book contained vast tracts of space separating a burned-out asteroid from a dying planet or two. Did I worry? Plenty.

Those were the years I hustled. Volunteered to cover the emergency room. Took calls for other doctors and filled in for them on vacations. Gave talks on the Elixir of Youth to senior citizens' groups.

If a doctor persists, as I have, in staying in one place for forty years with his smile and shoeshine intact, the patients will start appearing like kernels of popcorn exploding in hot oil—a few puffs at first, then a sudden dozen, and finally a white-headed swarm clambering to get out of the frying pan and into the fire. Catch them if you can! Bowl them over! Butter them up! (Take the aforementioned with a grain of salt.)

While we're on the subject, I would like to go on record as deploring the demise of movie popcorn. Plastic bags of pre-popped corn are delivered to movie theaters in the dead of night like corpses being dropped off at the morgue.

Husks of their former selves, these stale dry puffs are dumped into a glass box and heated with a light bulb. This dead-white mound under glass lies in a state similar to that of my childhood heroine, Snow White. Alas, no Prince Charming for *this* Snow White! Instead, a common usher, pressed into service behind the refreshment stand, bestows a final kiss of death on the remains by purporting to "butter" them. We popcorn freaks, of course, pay extra for this slick version of an otherwise tasteless pulp.

It may be a sign of the times, but it seems to me that neither my patients nor my popcorn are what they used to be twenty years ago.

Rule 38

When She's Absolutely, Positively Sure She Isn't Pregnant, Get a Pregnancy Test

---

OF ALL THE DIAGNOSES I've missed, one of the most elusive is pregnancy. Maybe it's because pregnancy isn't a disease, but it often brings symptoms that look like one. You wouldn't think such a commonly experienced human phenomenon could be mislabeled as intestinal flu, would you? Or chronic fatigue? Or joggers' nipples? Well, let me tell you, it's been called worse: exogenous obesity, acute agitated depression, self-induced vomiting. I could go on, but my self-esteem rebels.

The first person a woman in my practice sees when she becomes pregnant is me, her dumb male internist. Her major complaint is fatigue, which narrows the diagnostic possibilities to ten thousand. *Of course* she had a period last month. Well, maybe it wasn't as heavy as usual. She has used her diaphragm with fail-safe precautions more stringent than those enforced in a missile silo. Her breasts are a little sore, but she jogs a lot. Morning sickness? The night before, she had barbecued ribs, french fries, jalapeño peppers, and butter brickle ice cream—*ad nauseum*? Of course. Pregnant? No way.

The physical exam in early pregnancy is no help—I've never seen such normal women. (Unless she has an ectopic pregnancy and I'm able to feel a swollen, tender fallopian tube.)

Most of the time my patient and I sit looking at one another after the examination, wondering what she is doing in a doctor's office. For lack of anything better to offer, I suggest a pregnancy test. She demurs. The last time she had intercourse? "What decade is this, doctor?" I persist. The test, needless to say, is positive. Hail, Mary. I refer her to an obstetrician and take a Xanax.

I'm reminded of other veiled diagnoses a doctor can't afford to miss. A middle-aged man is about to have coronary bypass surgery. His kidney function tests are borderline-high. His prostate is a little enlarged, but what fifty-six-year-old man's isn't? Am I possibly sending this man into heart surgery with blocked kidneys? I say what the hell and get a renal sonogram. The patient's chronically obstructed kidneys are the size and shape of a movie producer's swimming pool. I call in a urologist and take a Xanax.

For the first time in her life a sixty-year-old woman is having diarrhea. She is dressed in seven layers of haute couture, and rather than wade through all that finery to do a rectal exam, I prescribe Kaopectate. A week later she still has diarrhea. The by-now unavoidable rectal exam shows a gigantic fecal impaction—eighteen layers of haute cuisine—that has probably been there a month. Two hours, twelve sets of rubber gloves, and four tubes of lubricant later, she is cured and I'm much older and a little wiser.

Rule 39

Create the Illusion of Being Less Stressed than Your Patients

---

IF A YOUNG DOCTOR wants to live to see his fortieth birthday, he's going to have to learn to mold the gelatin of his emotions into a semblance of the Rock of Gibraltar. He mustn't let depressed patients drag him down to their niche in the pits or let nervous patients yank him up into their electrical thunderheads. He must be the eye in the storm of his patients.

To survive private practice, I have learned to close my eyes to meditation, to turn my back to massage.

I borrow heavily from other medical cultures. To get me though a bad week in the office, I rely on massage and meditation, as well as Bombay gin—but not all at once, as a rule.

I meditate twenty minutes twice a day (before and after work) and have a massage on Sundays at the Church of Saints Supine & Prone. I pump my Schwinn exercise bike thirty minutes on Tuesday, Thursday, and Saturday mornings. I drink three ounces of gin no more than five days a week.

If you like to drink, as I do, I urge you to buy a measuring glass and titrate your own dose of ethanol as carefully as a diabetic pulling insulin into his syringe. The two days of abstinence allow the damaged liver and brain cells a chance to recover before they are hit by the next tsunami of firewater.

If you stroll through the hallways of the René Descartes University in Paris, you will observe the bronze busts of the great physicians of France. Knowing the Gallic penchant for *spiritus frumenti*, I suspect that many of these fabled *docteurs* were plastered long before they were bronzed. In the same tradition, an American doc on high doses of booze erects a plaster-of-paris bust of himself each night at the dinner table. It is his family who must drag the completed work—the feet of clay, the knees of wax, the torso of veined marble—off to bed.

Managing one's own stresses is the toughest part of practicing medicine. Harry Truman said, "If you can't stand the heat, get out of the kitchen." Even Harry was not immune to the soothing powers of bourbon and seven-card stud. Besides, he had Bess in the kitchen.

Rule 40

If You Drink, Don't Drive; If You Smoke, Don't Bother Wearing Your Seat Belt

AFTER FORTY YEARS OF private practice, the achievement of which I'm most proud is having helped two hundred or so patients quit smoking. I am positively evangelical on the subject of smoking, having quit a three-pack-a-day habit the morning I opened my office. (Of course, I *never* inhaled.) When I start talking cigarettes, the hurricane force of my outrage turns the glow at the end of a butt to ash—the Joe Blow at the other end of the butt into a born-again nonsmoker.

My favorite punch line is to tell a smoker she's microwaving herself to death: She looks like a million bucks on the outside, a charred ruin on the inside.

As a physician, I'm sick to think that part of my income tax goes to subsidize the tobacco industry. Of course, another part goes to sustain the moral fiber of the Surgeon General, who, through the smoke of this particular battle, warns us that "Smoking Causes Lung Cancer, Heart Disease, Emphysema, and May Complicate Pregnancy." In page after page of print ads, these remarks appear in a small black-bordered rectangular box that is dwarfed by an infinite expanse of golf course.

If I, Captain Oscar London, U.S. Army Medical Corps, ret., were ever called back, Cincinnatus-like, to serve my country as Surgeon

General, I'd put the smiling golfer in the small black-bordered rectangular box (as a reminder of his imminent funeral) and devote the remaining space to my warning:

THE SURGEON GENERAL HAS DETERMINED THAT THE ONLY SMOKERS WHO DON'T INHALE ARE DEAD SMOKERS.

It's almost as if the tobacco industry had calibrated the dose of its product to sustain the buying power of the smoker for thirty-five years. By contrast, the dying power of lung cancer is an unprofitable six months—*but* victims of emphysema and chronic bronchitis sometimes survive for fifteen two-pack-a-day years, which can guarantee marginal profitability for the tobacco company while the ad agencies penetrate the teenage market. The sudden market dropout of a smoker from heart disease, of course, has to be written off as a dead loss.

Rule 41

If You Think You're Indispensable, Check Your Appointment Book a Week after You Drop Dead

---

DEATH, AS I TELL my medical students, is as inevitable as a fat redhead at a motorcyclist's funeral. You've seen her on the eleven o'clock news. Her twelve-pound necklace of turquoise and silver clanks with each sob. Plump tears stain her blue denim vest. But once the remains of her lover and his inseparable bike have been lowered into the pit, she hops with alacrity onto the back of her new boyfriend's Kawasaki. She clutches him for dear life about his waist and the two of them roar off happily ever after.

When a doctor dies, the fickle redhead symbolizes all that remains of his practice. His instant successor is that hotshot on the Kawasaki.

The late doctor's picture in the obituary column was taken twenty years ago; no one recognizes him. Some genuine tears are shed by his family, twelve patients, seven pharmacists, and his office landlord. In a week the dearly departed is an anecdote: "Doc London? Dead? Oh yeah, he used to be my sister-in-law's doctor until she broke out in that penicillin rash."

Patients lose respect for a doctor who has died before they have. Those whose appointments have to be canceled as a consequence of what he's done are furious with him. They'd sue him for malpractice if he could be stood up in court.

Even the World's Best Doctor has no illusions that his good works will survive him for long. I think it's entirely healthy for a doctor to know he isn't indispensable. It keeps him from playing God too seriously.

If I should take up the motorcycle in my declining years, I would want the fat redhead to say at my graveside, "The doctor is dead. Long live the patients."

Rule 42

Beware of Sharing Coffee with Young Ladies or Quaffing Sherry with Old Ones

IT SOUNDS HARMLESS ENOUGH at first. Before leaving your office after an upbeat visit, the young lady says brightly, "Why don't we have a cup of coffee sometime?"

Or the elderly lady says, "Why don't you drop by for a glass of sherry?"

Under these circumstances, a cup of coffee and a glass of sherry are the most dangerous potions a doctor can drink.

The first cup of coffee is in a restaurant; lots of laughs, loads of eye contact. The second cup of coffee is in her apartment; fewer laughs, different contact. The third cup of coffee is allowed to sit on the end table and grow cold. At the bottom of the seventeenth cup of coffee are grounds for a lawsuit.

The first glass of sherry is in her lovely home; lots of childhood anecdotes, loads of old photographs. Your respectful visit is the most exciting thing that's happened to her in thirty years. Out of restiveness, you keep bolting glass after glass of sherry. Each time, she pours you a refill from seemingly inexhaustible reserves.

Unwittingly, your gallant social call, combined with the sherry *she* has been downing, have aroused in her ardent expectations of awesome proportions. When you are allowed to finally stagger to the door, it is only on condition that you return the following week for "another glass of sherry." The prospect conjures up visions of drowning in a wine-dark sea.

The night before your next glass of sherry, you dream that you are Jacques Cousteau, scuba diving in twelve fathoms of amontillado. Suddenly a great white shark with dentures takes a shine to you and chomps through your air hose.

I, for one, think of courtrooms and Cousteau whenever I'm asked to share coffee or quaff sherry.

Rule 43

Avoid Hospital Meetings like the Plague

SOME DOCTORS HAVE A talent for administration, a passion for bureaucracy—a deeply felt longing to sit down with their fellow man and a tuna fish sandwich and discuss, at length, whether the sign outside Intensive Care should read Do Not Enter or Authorized Personnel Only.

I have a Kafkaesque revulsion to meetings. I'd rather be stood up before a firing squad than be seated with a hospital committee. A firing squad, at least, is a group of men who don't lounge around and shilly-shally. What's more, the chairman of a firing squad doesn't appoint a Subcommittee on Blindfolds & Cigarettes before he adjourns the brief session with an unambiguous "Fire!"

As I see it, a doctor's place is in the office or at the patient's bedside, not in Conference Room E. I will go to any length to avoid serving on a hospital committee. Some years ago, I let it be bruited about the hospital corridors that I was undergoing outpatient care for a mild case of Hansen's disease.* For a blissful three years I was not asked to serve on a hospital committee. In fact, my peers appointed a subcommittee to make sure I didn't go *near* a conference room.

*Aka leprosy.

Rule 44

Don't Underestimate the Healing Power of Blarney

I NEVER LET A patient leave my office before I dispense at least a homeopathic dose of flattery. I give an acutely wounded ego a booster shot of blarney the moment he shuffles through the door. "You look wonderful, Morris! You haven't aged in five years!" (This to a man who has aged ten years since his mistress ran off with his business partner a week ago.)

I make a point of greeting a female patient before she exchanges her clothes for a paper gown: she may have taken pains to look well-dressed for the doctor. After she's wrapped and tied herself in paper, I remark, "You look terrific in white."

There's no stopping me. I might say something nice about a lady's bracelet or ring or a man's cufflinks or even his crown jewels. Actually, during the course of a routine genital exam, I matter-of-factly remark, "Perfectly normal," if I sense a man may be self-conscious about his sexual endowment. To tell the truth, the normal range of size in this closely guarded sector of the male anatomy is somewhere between a Sidewinder and a Titan missile—so "perfectly normal" describes the armamentarium of almost any man.

I have never succeeded in killing a patient with an overdose of flattery.

Rule 45

Call in Death as a Consultant

I INVITE DEATH INTO my office as a consultant on every patient I examine. He sits there, as I see him, in the black uniform and spit-polished boots of an SS Colonel, a white Death's Head insignia perched above the visor of his cap. Through rimless glasses that flash in my examining lights, he studies every move I make. For example, I forget to ask a patient with borderline hypertension to come back in six months to have me recheck his blood pressure. Death, seated at attention, scratches a few words in his black notebook.

A patient with vague chest pains and a slightly abnormal EKG resists my advice that he go into the hospital for observation. The SS Colonel smiles expectantly while the patient pleads with me to go home. After the patient thanks me profusely and escapes the office, the Colonel tears a page from his notebook and jumps up. With a click of his heels, Death hands me a Certificate.

I like to tell medical students that a doctor is only as effective as the consultants he picks. Death, I have found, is the most accommodating of consultants. He will even make housecalls, especially when I won't.

Rule 46

Don't Be a Semi-Pro

A PRO IS SOMEONE who works when he's sick and is told how marvelous he looks. A pro gives a high-energy performance up to the final curtain, whether it's drawn across a stage or around a bed. In sickness and in health. I haven't missed a scheduled day of work in over twenty years. (*Applause, cheers, whistles.*) Solo practice has been a good incentive for me to stay in shape. Getting run-down and sick, I have found, is not the best professional stance a physician can take—unless, of course, he suffers a coronary occlusion: the only illness in which a doctor can take professional pride. (That much of a pro I hope never to be.)

Ever since I learned that grandmasters in chest keep their professional edge by jogging before a match, I've tried to follow in their footsteps. (I can run circles around Gary Kasporov.) For a life of the mind, it helps to have the body of an athlete. I was born with the body of a queen's rook, but have trained it to resemble a king's knight, with a potbelly. No stranger to the Round Table, I am known as Sir Lunch-a-lot.

In an effort to stay in the ranks of the pros, I preach my anti-smoking sermon, after forty years, with all the old fire and brimstone. A medical pro must be able to listen with a straight face to every complaint a patient makes, even if she says she suffers from "fireballs of the Uticas" when she means fibroids of the uterus.

As a final professional touch, a doctor, I believe, should try to project at least a little magic—something that left medicine when the shaman took off his feathered headdress and put on a Littman stethoscope. Quite a few patients want to believe their doctor is not only brilliant but has a white rabbit and a string of silk handkerchiefs somewhere inside that black bag of his. Not *my* patients of course—they'd point out that they're allergic to rabbit fur and would prefer a Kleenex to a silk hanky. Some of my patients will tell you the only magic I'm capable of is making their money disappear. It's hard enough for me to be a doctor, let along a magician, but I try.

A professional magician, you'll note, dresses impeccably, has an air of supreme confidence, a flair for the dramatic, and is not without some humor. When he saws the pretty lady in half, she comes out whole. I leave that particular trick to my fast-handed colleagues in surgery. For me, I'd like you to pick a disease, any disease, but don't tell me what it is.

I am not a semi-pro. I have always tried to act the role of the doctor I hope someday to be.

Rule 47

Pick Up the Phone like Itzhak Perlman Picking Up a Strad

TELEPHONES AND EGGS BENEDICT are the leading causes of premature death among doctors. Since eggs Benedict are avoidable, I will confine my remarks to telephones—those most necessary of medical evils.

To tell the truth, I encourage my patients to call me. As a result of my open-phone policy, there's a constant ringing in my office not unlike the din of church bells in Russia after Napoleon's retreat from Moscow.

I have drilled my receptionist to take every call in stride and to ask each patient, unless it's an emergency, to let me phone back later. The average half-life of a receptionist in my office is four months. After about the twelve-hundredth phone call, it is necessary for me to bind and gag her and drive her to the nearest crisis intervention center. A few days of primal screaming and massive sedation, and she's ready to pick up the phone again and say "Dr. London's office, will you hold please?"

My own telephone manner is styled to gather maximum information in the shortest possible time with minimal blood loss. The first thing I do is take a deep breath before speaking. This prevents my voice from strangling itself to an inaudible whisper, whereupon the patient can leap in and capture the conversation for as long as *his* breath holds out (which, in a nonsmoker, I've clocked up to one-half hour).

Another strategy that works for me is to assume the telephone is a time bomb rigged to go off if I don't hang up the receiver in three minutes. This technique imparts a tone of urgency to my voice, which most patients correctly interpret as a desire for them to shut up soon or else. If an insensitive caller continues to talk, a loud recording of my voice cuts in:

"This is Dr. London. Thanks to your deadly monologue, I can no longer continue this conversation; you have talked me into an early grave. At the sound of the explosive tone, please leave your name and phone number. As the prime suspect in my death, you have the right to remain silent. Anything you say can and will be used against you. You are permitted one phone call to your lawyer. God help him."

Rule 48

When a Patient Rejects You, Rejoice

THERE MUST BE SOME mistake! This isn't happening! The small rectangle of paper bears a rival colleague's letterhead and is signed by one of my oldest and dearest patients. She is leaving me for another shaman! Oh God! Stabbed in the back! How could she *do* this to me?

I've long since given up trying to figure out why any patient would choose to defect from the practice of the World's Best Doctor. I simply choke back a sob and promptly send her new doctor—the poor bastard—a summary of my records on the errant patient. If the patient herself doesn't tell me, I don't try to find out why she bolted. As long as her request for a transfer is not followed by an envelope embossed with the name of a law firm, I rejoice. I smile like a mule chewing briars when I think of the misery she may have saved me by transferring her baggage of woe to another doctor's doorstep. Besides, she used to steal my *New Yorkers*.

Rule 49

Orchestrate Your Patients, Unless You're Ready for Your Requiem

9:57 A.M. DR. LONDON arrives at his office a few minutes before his first patient's appointment. Cradling the cup of coffee his receptionist has prepared for him, he steps into his consultation room, locks the door, and sits down. Fifteen minutes later, his receptionist buzzes him on the intercom to suggest that he start his day's work. There is no answer.

10:31 A.M. Inspector Holmes arrives, accompanied by his principal cocaine supplier and good friend, Dr. Watson. They force the consultation room door to find Dr. London slumped over his desk. Dead.

"A coronary, by the looks of it," blurts out Dr. Watson, whose appearances before the Credentials Committee of St. Bartholomew's have become increasingly frequent in recent years.

"Not at all, Watson," says Holmes, bending over the corpse. "No crease in the earlobe, no arcus senilis, no nicotine stains on the fingers. Regard, if you will, the bulging calf muscles of an exercyclist. No, Watson, your unfortunate colleague here is not the victim of coronary occlusive disease."

"I say, Holmes, look at this—obviously the work of a vampire."

Watson points to a pair of bluish puncture wounds, an inch part, on the left side of Dr. London's neck.

"Hmmmm," intones Holmes, perusing the tiny wounds with his Bausch & Lomb magnifying glass. "Ineffectual, self-inflicted ballpoint pen wounds."

"You amaze me, Holmes," says Watson. "But how did the doctor die?"

"Elementary, my dear Watson," replies Holmes, studying a slip of paper on which the victim's head had been resting. "Oh, Miss Wigglesworth," says Holmes, "would you be so kind as to step in here for a moment?"

Trembling, the late doctor's receptionist approaches the scene of the crime.

"Are you responsible for scheduling each day's appointments?" asks Holmes.

"Y-yes, sir."

"You will note, Miss Wigglesworth, that your late employer, Dr. London, scratched an exclamation mark with his ballpoint pen after the names of the first three patients."

The receptionist bolts for the door but is tripped up by the crook of Dr. Watson's cane. She lies whimpering on the floor as Holmes wraps up the case.

"Surely you knew when you scheduled Mrs. Van Hippschtein, Mr. Carrowaddy, and Miss Krochmalnick *sequentially*, that your doctor would never survive seeing them *one after the other*."

"It served the bastard right," hisses the receptionist. "Not one bloody raise in four years!"

"So you see, Watson," explains the inspector as the two men make their ways to Holmes's afternoon violin lesson, "when the late Dr. London saw that he would have to face three of his most depressed and demanding patients *consecutively*, he attempted to take his life by stabbing himself with a cheap ballpoint pen given to him by a pharmaceutical representative.

"When this attempt failed, he glanced once more at his appointments and died of a massive overdose of self-pity. He had chagrin written all over his face."

(Indeed, Watson had been so engrossed with the victim's neck wounds that he failed to see the word *chagrin* scrawled in ballpoint ink on the late doctor's cheeks and forehead.)

"Good heavens, Holmes," exclaims Dr. Watson, "to think that an appointment book in the hands of the wrong receptionist can be a lethal weapon!"

Rule 50

Drive Wooden Stakes through the Hearts of Financial Advisors

THE WORLD'S BEST DOCTOR is the World's Worst Businessman. I am the willing victim of financial vampires who, by day, cling upside down from the leaking ceilings of tax shelters. By night, they form a holding pattern outside my office window, waiting to swoop in one by one.

These fat bats are only too happy to "drop by your office some night after work to discuss a matter of great importance to someone in your tax bracket."

With your collar loosened and your sleeves rolled up—it is after hours, after all—you welcome into your office a black-garbed figure who is rather long in the tooth. He hands you his business card, and you fail to notice that his home office is based in Transylvania. Against your better judgment, you stick your neck out.

Three months later, your colleagues remark how pale you look. Your dentist suggests filing down your incisors to correct a sudden overbite you seem to have developed. When you step into your lofty tax shelter of oil lease-backs, you discover that you are up to your knees in bat guano.

I can't tell you how many thousands of green corpuscles these Draculoids have drained from my savings account through the years.

Suffice it to say that ten years ago the annual report on my cattle-feed venture featured a photograph of six hundred steers lying belly-up on a snow-clad hillside in Montana. The caption, as I recall, mentioned something about bovine burcellosis and bankruptcy.

Five years ago, just before harvest time, my two-acre grove of pistachio trees in Orange County was stripped bare by a renegade pack of chimpanzees who had escaped from the San Diego Zoo. The chimps finally settled in Silicon Valley where they formed a computer company on whose common stock I lost a bundle.

Six months ago I persuaded a cardiac surgeon who works in our hospital to go public. He was just starting practice, needed some upfront cash, and had terrific growth potential. Meyer Kornbleet, MD, Inc.—a glamour issue. I bought two hundred and fifty shares on margin of Meyer Kornbleet Preferred. In a week his stock split, and so did Meyer Kornbleet, with his blonde secretary, to Acapulco. On his return, Mrs. Kornbleet liquidated Meyer Kornbleet, MD, Inc., with a small acquisition from Smith & Wesson.

My financial advice to young doctors: Try to make a living in the office rather than a killing in the stock market. Also, close your office windows after sunset.

Rule 51

Exhume Old Records and Postpone Your Patient's Burial

JAMES PARKER WAS FLUNKING his fourth year of medical school. A tall, handsome young man with thinning flaxen hair, Jim wanted desperately to be a doctor. The death of his mother and father in a car wreck during his second year of medical school, and the break-up of his marriage during his third, had combined to keep Jim's head in his hands instead of his books.

I was a resident physician in a century-old teaching hospital and Jim was assigned to my ward. His grades in the basic sciences, after an early freshman peak, had been abysmal. His only chance for squeaking through medical school was to shine in his clinical work. As his mentor, I knocked myself out trying to make him into an effective clinician, but it was like trying to breathe life into a zombie.

Jim's final grade in his fourth year, his only hope for graduating, hinged on how well he could present to the chairman of the Department of Medicine a case he had worked up from scratch. The chairman, Professor Marcus Cohen, was probably the brightest internist in the country; he had a withering contempt for medical students who failed to live up to his Olympian standards.

The case Jim chose was that of a sixty-two-year-old woman whose chest X-ray showed a coin lesion in her right lung—a round lump possibly representing a curable cancer. She didn't recall having a previous X-ray for comparison.

She smoked two packs of cigarettes a day, had severe angina and mild congestive heart failure. She was at obvious risk to undergo chest surgery to see if the coin lesion was cancerous. I reluctantly consented to have a hotshot thoracic surgeon put her on his schedule for an open-lung biopsy in a week. Meanwhile, I had to help Jim prepare the case for presentation.

Had Jim been my own son, I couldn't have worked harder drilling in on every nuance of the case. I even doubled as his voice coach, trying to stir up a little fire in his delivery of the facts.

The patient, already sick and tired, grew more so at the sight of Jim and me approaching her bed for yet another rehearsal of her medical history. I even voice-coached *her*; the chairman of the Department of Medicine did not suffer lightly patients who mumbled during Grand Rounds.

On the day before Jim was to present her to the chairman, I asked the patient once again. "Mrs. Connery, are you sure you never had a chest X-ray before, for any reason?"

Above her head, I could see a 15-watt bulb light up.

"O dear Lord," she said, in the heightened voice my coaching had achieved, "I think they took lots of X-rays in this same dump when I was kicked by a milk-wagon horse—about thirty years ago."

"But we looked through your old X-ray file and found nothing," I said.

"Were you married then, Mrs. Connery?" Jim asked.

The patient's cheeks flushed with anger.

"Yeah, I was married then," she said. "To Ed Muldoon—that bastard. He was my second—no my third—husband. That's right. My second husband was Ralph-the-Flasher. He once flashed an under-cover cop, but got off due to 'insufficient evidence.'"

A fit of wet coughing interrupted her mirthless laughter.

At the mention of her third-husband-the-bastard's name, I knew my medical student had a chance to be his mother's son-the-doctor. I grabbed Jim by the wrinkled shoulders of his white jacket and shook him.

"Don't tell a soul," I said. "Just go down to the file room and find her old films, under Kathleen Muldoon. Find them even if it kills you."

The X-ray vault in the ancient city hospital would have made the Black Hole of Calcutta look like a tanning studio in Los Angeles. Tens of thousands of mouldering X-rays were stacked in perpetual gloom on the grimy shelves. Jim spent fourteen hours searching by flash-light for the buried chest film of Kathleen Connery, the former Mrs. Ed ("The Bastard") Muldoon.

Just after three in the morning, five hours before his presen-tation, Jim shook me awake in the residents' quarters. My eyes snapped open to behold a large battered envelope tremulously lit by Jim's flashlight.

We had to pry apart the decaying films inside; it was almost as if they had clung to one another for protection in that dank and dingy vault. At last, we found the old chest film. Through scratches and smudges we could see our patient's coin lesion, unchanged in size for more than thirty years—and therefore not cancer! It was probably the calcified remains of an old infection. Jim had saved the patient a major operation that might very well have killed her.

James Parker was fully prepared to meet Professor Marcus Cohen, who in turn was fully prepared to flunk him. Shakily at first, my protégé set up the story as a routine case of coin lesion that demanded surgical excision.

As expected, Professor Cohen asked, "Are there any old films for comparison?"

"I was sure there weren't," I said, interrupting. "But Parker dug all night in the file room and look what he found."

With a magician's flourish, the medical student slapped the ancient film on the view box, ripping the X-ray in half! But rent asunder or not, the film clearly showed the old coin lesion, a piece of buried diagnostic gold.

"No surgery for this lady!" concluded James Parker.

Seated in a wheelchair, Mrs. Connery revealed a clue to her complex medical history: a dazzling smile. Professor Cohen, a bald-headed bantam in a long white coat, jumped to his feet and shook Jim's hand. (Nothing delights an internist more than robbing a surgeon of a case.)

The medical student is now Dr. James Parker, an internist in St. Louis—remarried, with two children, the first of whom he named Oscar. Poor kid.

Rule 52

Remember a Malpractice Lawyer in Your Prayers

Dear Lord,

Bless my family and friends and cause the teeth of a malpractice lawyer to falleth like hailstones in the marble hallways of justice. O Lord, may the next passage of the litigator's comb through his silver locks snatcheth him bald. May the jury he turneth to face on the morrow behold that lo, he failed to zippeth up his fly. May his bowels turneth to concrete at home and to water in the courtroom. When he goeth to switch on the ignition, may his large German vehicle droppeth its transmission like unto a cow giving birth. May the next doctor he chargeth with malpractice sueth the lawyer in turn for malpractice and collecteth mightily, and then some, for ever and ever. Amen.

Rule 53

Let the Patient Make His Own Diagnosis

TRADE SECRET: THE BEST diagnosticians in medicine are not internists, but patients. If only the doctor would sit down, shut up, and listen, the patient will eventually tell him the diagnosis.

During my brief stint in the Army Medical Corps, I spent six months conducting sick call for a peacetime location of one thousand men. The sergeant who ushered the patients into the long hallway outside my office did not subscribe to the germ theory of disease. Sergeant Hotchkiss invented his own differential diagnosis: any soldier on sick call without an open, bleeding wound was either a Goof-off or a Fuck up. A typical morning would begin with Hotchkiss reporting to me, "Sir, I got five Goof-offs and a Fuck-up dying to see you."

One day, just before lunch, Sergeant Hotchkiss came down heavily on a young private who complained that his feet cramped on a long march. Through my closed door I heard Hotchkiss bark, "Well, whose feet in hell *don't* cramp on a long march?" Hotchkiss, during this phase of his career, was not bucking for either the Nobel Peace Prize or the Nobel Prize in Medicine.

The private entered my office apologetically. When I asked him what his trouble was, he blushed and said his feet always cramped on a long march. Standing behind him, Hotchkiss silently mouthed the diagnosis: "Fuck-up."

"Did your feet ever cramp before you enlisted?" I asked.

"Yessir, lotsa times. My doc back home couldn't figure it out. He said there probably wasn't enough blood gettin' down to my feet."

Hotchkiss interrupted at this point to remind me that lunch hour had struck. Asking myself what Douglas MacArthur would do, I looked up and said, "Sergeant, I'll be quite a while with this patient. We'll break for lunch when I'm finished."

I could see Hotchkiss beginning to enter the early phases of Spam withdrawal. He responded to my announcement with the ultimate weapon of the outraged non-com: a slow, solemn salute of surpassing diameter and grace—as difficult to master as a perfect first serve in tennis.

Alone with the patient, I resumed my inquiry.

"Did your doctor back home find anything else wrong with you?"

"Yep. He said I had high blood pressure. I don't see how I passed the army physical. Guess they was so rushed they just passed me through."

Before I had even asked the patient to strip down to his shorts, he had already handed me the diagnosis: coarctation of the aorta. Sure enough, his blood pressure was sky-high, he had a loud heart murmur, and I couldn't feel any pulsations in his legs.

Three weeks later the patient was cured of his potentially fatal disease by an aortic bypass operation at taxpayers' expense. The World's Best Doctor had made his first major-league diagnosis by shutting up a sergeant and listening to a private.

Rule 54

Don't Turn Your Back on Back Pain; Don't Airily Dismiss a Complaint of Gas

WHEN CERTAIN PATIENTS WALK through the front door of my office, I run out the back door. Some clinical problems defeat even the World's Best Doctor. Obesity and alcoholism, for example, trounce me every time. (Weight Watches and Alcoholics Anonymous do an infinitely better job that I do in reshaping the bodies and minds of overeaters and substance abusers of every stripe.)

Of course, if you get in the habit of referring *all* your difficult problems for treatment elsewhere, you will end up with a practice devoted exclusively to the care of sore throats and mild anxiety. I, for one, do not turn my back on back pain nor airily dismiss a complaint of gas. In fact, back pain and gas are two of my favorite challenges.

Having been knifed in the back myself once by an acute lumbar sprain, I am Dr. Sympathy himself when it comes to treating a fellow sufferer. In a word, my heart goes out to those whose backs go out.

In my experience, lumbar ligament pain and slipped disc are the major causes of acute low back pain. An X-ray doesn't throw much light on the problem but should be done to rule out nightmares like bone cancer and osteoporotic fractures.

Whether the cause is ligament sprain (common) or slipped disc (uncommon), the treatment for severe back pain is the same: complete bed rest for one day—not getting up, except to be helped to the bathroom. (Bed rest is to low back pain what penicillin is to the streptococcus.) One day down. To sustain life while his back mends, the prostrate victim should be thrown a sandwich from time to time by a loving hand or a hired one.

During this day the patient has a choice of two positions: flat on his back or curled up on his side like a cat. (I've yet to hear a cat bellyache about low back pain.) *Sitting up is forbidden*. (Sitting up is to low back pain what bourbon is to alcoholism.)

A heating pad may help, provided it's turned to the lowest setting. (The back is already in enough trouble without being grilled medium-rare.) For a ligament sprain, I often inject the iliac crest on the affected side with lidocaine and a corticosteroid. Every now and then, this technique works so well that after the day of bed rest the patient will do handsprings to express his rapture. He then has to be carried back to bed for a repeat confinement.

If the patient is still in agony, even after a couple more days of bed rest, I put him in a corset and gently pack him off to a physical therapist. (On the packing crate I mark THIS SIDE UP and HANDLE WITH CARE.)

Two weeks later, if the patient reappears bent over at my front door, I go out the back door. Before I slam it, I leave word with my receptionist to give the patient the name of the best orthopedist or neurosurgeon in town.

The patient with gas is about as miserable as the one with back pain and equally difficult to treat. If the patient doesn't come right out and tell you he suffers from gas, you can pretty well make the diagnosis by looking up and noting that he seems to be bobbing gently against the ceiling. I refer, of course, to the extreme case.

Rather than tell the agonized patient he must learn to sail through life like a hot-air balloon, I make every effort to rid him of his trapped vapors. I teach him to breathe out before he swallows. For a week I forbid the following: carbonated drinks, milk, beans, onions, cabbage, whole grains, and excessive carbohydrates, especially fruit. If this elimination diet fails and the patient is still hovering Hindenburg-like above my exam table, the next step is to displace his gas with barium. For the patient over fifty, the doctor must make sure the gas is not a sign of gastrointestinal cancer.

If a thorough GI workup proves, like the diet I prescribed, fruitless, I expose my trump card—psyllium. This magic powder turns to a gelatinous blob when mixed with water and, in my opinion, is the greatest medication in gastroenterology. It not only banishes gas but controls diarrhea and constipation due to a spastic bowel. It may even prevent cancer of the colon as a bonus. A tablespoon of psyllium powder is not the greatest-tasting substance in the world but neither is a handful of bran, which it resembles in effect.

Ever since I became known around town as the doc who cures back pain and gas, a Macy's parade of stooped marchers accompanied by inflated objects overhead has made the pilgrimage to my office. Sometimes the price of success is more than anyone can afford.

Rule 55

Ask Your Patient What's Shaking Down at Work and What's Cooking at Home

LONDON'S LAW: If a patient is miserable at work *and* at home, he will come down with a major physical ailment.

This double-whammied patient is easy to diagnose: stroke, heart attack, peptic ulcer, to name a few classics.

LONDON'S FIRST CORRELATE: If a patient is miserable in just *one* place—at home or at work—he will bring in a list of symptoms as long as the table of contents in Cecil's *Medicine*, and no diagnosis will be up to the task. Only partially burned out, this patient is en route to a major physical ailment.

LONDON'S SECOND CORRELATE: If a person is content at work *and* at home, he will never darken a doctor's doorway.

With every patient I see, I try to find out what's shaking down at work, and what's cooking at home.

Many years back, I treated an elderly White Russian who had served as a general in the Czar's army and was now trying to make it as a real estate broker in Nixon's America. Whenever he failed to make a sale, which was often, he had to restrain himself from taking down his jeweled sword from the wall behind his desk and running the client through. Boy, did he have symptoms! (A recurrent, stabbing pain in the abdomen, of course, was one.) Fortunately, he also had an excellent marriage.

His wife had been a lady-in-waiting to the Czarina, spoke five languages poetically, and had grown more beautiful with each passing decade. She could cook a bowl of *pelmeni* whose aroma caused everyone downwind to hum something from Rachmaninoff. Beleaguered at work, the General had formidable reinforcements at home.

One afternoon, his wife dragged the General—pale and groaning—into my office and demanded that he be hospitalized.

"How's business?" I asked.

"Never better," she said. "Last month he sold an apartment building for a small fortune. He was the happiest man in the world. Now look at him. Doctor, put Gregor in the hospital."

"How are things at home?" I asked.

"Fine, wonderful. *Doctor, put Gregor in the hospital.*"

Who was I to stand up to the Czarina's lady-in-waiting? How could I, a former captain in the U.S. Army Medical Corps, refuse to hospitalize a stricken general? My only problem was that I couldn't come up with an admitting diagnosis. According to London's Second Correlate, a man who was happy at home and at work had no business being dragged half-dead to my office.

When I asked the General to point to where he hurt, he feebly passed his right hand over his entire body. Wherever I touched him, he groaned. My examination was otherwise completely negative.

Bowing to imperial pressure, I admitted the General with a diagnosis of pandynia (pain all over).

A week passed. Prodigious amounts of blood, urine, and barium were shunted about in a vain effort to make a diagnosis. The General refused to eat. Intravenous fluids kept him just viable enough to moan. He was dying before my eyes, and I didn't have a diagnosis. The only thing keeping him alive, I concluded, was my failure to find out what was wrong with him.

On the General's eighth day of hospitalization, his son-in-law, Sergei, accosted me after work in my office garage and swore me to secrecy. Russian intrigue! In a hoarse whisper, Sergei said, "Get the cat."

"You want me to get a CAT scan?" I asked, knowing too well how helpful a patient's relatives could be in leading an inept doctor to the correct diagnosis.

"Not a CAT scan," he said. "Sasha the cat. Get rid of her."

It turned out that the patient's wife had adopted a stray cat the month before and had fallen madly in love with it. After glancing to the right and to the left, the son-in-law imitated the General's wife speaking to the cat in Russian baby talk. It was, admittedly, disgusting.

The General, accustomed to his wife's undiluted affection, reportedly went berserk with jealousy. It was beneath his regal dignity—and contrary to his military ethic—to admit that a cat without a pedigree was defeating him.

Recently triumphant at work, but acutely miserable at home, the General nondiagnostically fell apart. Had the bottom fallen out of the real estate market at the same time that Sasha invaded his home, he would, by London's Law, have gone on to suffer a conventional stroke, heart attack, or peptic ulcer. But a man dying from feline envy was beyond my diagnostic ken—or kennel; I should have called a vet to the General's bedside.

With the diagnosis in the bag, I gave the wife a choice: her husband or the cat. After a shocking amount of soul-searching, she gave up the cat.

Over the wireless went the message: SASHA EVICTED. When the General received this eleventh-hour bulletin, he sprang from his deathbed and marched home in triumph.

A week later, his wife was in my office with a list of symptoms as long as the Trans-Siberian Railway.

Rule 56

When All Else Fails, Get a Five-Hour Glucose Tolerance Test

HYPOGLYCEMIA IS THE LAST refuge of the neurotic. Symptoms of hypoglycemia include fatigue, nervousness, faintness, and excessive appetite—a veritable smorgasbord for the neurotic, hungering for a physical diagnosis.

My patient—a pale, bearded lawyer—bursts into my office waving a magazine article he has just read. "This is it!" he shouts. "This is me!" He reminds me of Neville Chamberlain ecstatically waving a copy of the Munich Pact and proclaiming, "Peace for our time."

"This is it!" repeats the patient. "This is me!"

"Let me guess," I say. "Hypoglycemia."

"Exactly!" he says, dumbfounded. "Why haven't you tested me for it before?"

"Because a five-hour glucose tolerance test hurts and it won't tell me what's wrong with you."

"I want it anyway."

Reluctantly, I agree to order a five-hour glucose tolerance test. I have found that nothing subdues a demanding patient more effectively than being stuck in the arm at least five times in five hours, *at his own insistence*. Along about the fourth hour my would-be hypoglycemic makes as if to swoon. An emergency Snickers is administered.

In my experience, the results of a five-hour glucose tolerance test on a patient who requests it are invariably normal. The lawyer is heartbroken, of course, until he stumbles on an article about borderline adrenal insufficiency.

I don't mean to suggest that reactive hypoglycemia doesn't exist. I myself, if I miss lunch, begin to tremble and feel giddy around four o'clock. In my office refrigerator, next to my vials of tetanus toxoid and pneumococcal vaccine, I stock six unit-doses of Mars bars.

Physician, heal thyself.

Rule 57

Rehearse Your Final Words

I MAY NOT BE in the greatest shape on my deathbed to utter the following zingers that I would love to pass on to those I've left behind. So, for now—and then—here are my last words:

Always get power steering.

Never give digoxin on Sunday.

Keep your kids off motorcycles, cigarettes, and booze.

Give insulin four times a day.

Drive a big car.

Keep out of jails, hospitals, and HMOs.

Oscar London Quotables

"A clear understanding of how much I don't know
about medicine is one of my great strengths."

"As magically as a kiss can transform certain frogs
into princes, a hug can change a patient into a plaintiff."

"Were I to make the mistake of looking at the next day's
office schedule, I myself would be tempted to run
screaming to the nearest airport."

"The Streetcar Named Disease is never on schedule and
has but one destination—the End of the Line."

"A good nurse, like a good loaf of bread,
is the staff of life, and the crustier the better."

"Knowing the Gallic penchant for *spiritus frumenti*, I suspect
that many of these fabled *docteurs* were plastered
long before they were bronzed."

"When I asked the General to point to where he hurt,
he feebly passed his right hand over his entire body.
Wherever I touched him, he groaned. My examination
was otherwise completely negative."